THE
COMPLETE
GUIDE TO
VEGETARIAN
CONVENIENCE
FOODS

What People Are Saying About This Book

"This is one of the most valuable books to come along in years. I have found nothing else to compare with the basic advice, the resources, and the helpful hints contained in Gail Davis' book. I couldn't put it down."

— Charles Attwood, M.D., F.A.A.P.
Author, Dr. Attwood's Low-Fat Prescription For Kids

"At last, a book for people who want to eat well, but don't have time to cook. Gail Davis has done a masterful job, sleuthing out ready-to-eat foods that are healthful and great tasting. I will be recommending it to all my students."

— Jennifer Raymond
Author, The Peaceful Palate

"This book is a quick guide that should be on your kitchen counter next to your grocery list and in your glove compartment as you head to the store. This book lets you make the change to healthier fare quickly and with confidence."

— Neil D. Barnard, M.D.
President, Physicians Committee for Responsible Medicine

"The real challenge for vegetarians, is the same as for meat-eaters: to eat healthful meals that are satisfying. Although vegetarians seem to simply have less options to achieve their dietary goals, writers like Gail Davis have changed that perception. Through Gail, we learn that vegetarians do not 'sacrifice' anything. It is the meat-eaters who are making the real sacrifice."

— Alec Baldwin
Actor

"*The Complete Guide to Vegetarian Convenience Foods* is a valuable resource for anyone looking for better health through convenience foods."

— John McDougall, M.D. and Mary McDougall
authors, The McDougall Program for a Healthy Heart

". . .Makes vegetarian eating as easy as pie. A couch potato's dream guide to eating healthy snacks and meals. It made me so hungry I had to race to the grocery store."

— Ingrid E. Newkirk
President, People for the Ethical Treatment of Animals

"*The Complete Guide to Vegetarian Convenience Foods* is the answer to a question I'm asked a thousand times a year: 'So, now what do I eat?' Read Gail Davis's book. It's terrific and I loved it!'

— Howard F. Lyman
President, International Vegetarian Union and author of Mad Cowboy

"This book is a must for people who would like to become vegetarian, but thought it was too complicated and time-consuming an endeavor. Mainstream food processors and retailers are now making hundreds of completely vegetarian food products that are delicious, nutritious, and easy to prepare. Davis has taken the next step by bringing these foods home to practicing vegans and transitioning vegetarians, alike."

— Alex Hershaft, Ph.D.
President, Farm Animal Reform Movement

"Finally, a guide that takes you by the hand to the best vegetarian food available on the market. It's a map, it's a menu, it's a must have for every wanna be and every experienced vegetarian."

— Kevin Nealon
Actor/Comedian

THE
COMPLETE
GUIDE TO
VEGETARIAN
CONVENIENCE
FOODS

Gail B. Davis

Foreword by Neal D. Barnard, M.D.

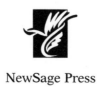

NewSage Press

THE COMPLETE GUIDE TO VEGETARIAN CONVENIENCE FOODS

Copyright © 1999 Gail B. Davis
Illustrations © 1999 Sylvia Walker

ISBN 0-939165-35-X

The views in this book are those of the author and not necessarily that of the publisher or of any other individual or organization. This book is designed to provide information; however, neither the author nor publisher are engaged in rendering nutritional counseling or medical advice. For these services, contact a professional in such matters.

The registered trademarks displayed in this book are the sole property of their respective owners.

Address Inquiries to:
NewSage Press
PO Box 607
Troutdale, OR 97060-0607
503-695-2211 fax: 503-695-5406

email: newsage@teleport.com
Web Site: http://www.teleport.com/~newsage

Book Cover Design by George Foster
Book Design by Nancy L. Doerrfeld-Smith; Production by Jenny Beranek

Printed in the United States on recycled paper with soy ink.

Distributed in the United States and Canada by
Publishers Group West 1-800-788-2123

Library of Congress Cataloging-in-Publication Data

Davis, Gail (Gail Barbara)
        The complete guide to vegetarian convenience food / by Gail B.
Davis; foreword by Neal Barnard.
        p. cm.
        Includes bibliographical references and index.
        ISBN 0-939165-35-X (alk. paper)
        1. Vegetarian cookery. 2. Convenience foods. I. Title.
TX837.D276   1999
641.5'636--dc21   99-20236
                                                           CIP

1 2 3 4 5 6 7 8 9 10

Dedication

To my mother, Edie Davis
for her unwavering
love and confidence in me.

Acknowledgments

For all of their love, support, encouragement, kindness, and faith in me, I would like to extend my most heartfelt appreciation to my dearest friends and associates, Parandeh Amini, Robert Baker, M.D., Howard Lyman, Jennifer Raymond and Stephen Avis, Alex Hershaft, Ph.D., Simon Oswitch, Stan Jensen, Pma Tregenza, Merrill Tilker, Justin and Barbara Kolb, Sandra Soule, Kannan Nadarajan, Roger Jacobson, Sophia Avants, Tania Soussan, Ray Watt, Elena McCaffrey, Ingrid Sherman, and Cherie Soria.

For their unique ideas and contributions of time, energy, and talent, many special thanks to Linda Nealon, Neal Barnard, M.D., Sylvia Walker, George Foster, Chiu-Nan Lai, David Morgan, Joe Sabah, Amina Lozada, Jeff and Sabrina Nelson, Greg Lemire, Jay Highman, Gary, Vina, and staff at Lassen Family Foods in Goleta, California, and Benjamin, Ken, Mark, and all of the outstanding librarians at the Santa Barbara Public Library.

Special thanks to the ever-nurturing Patti Breitman, the best cheering section anyone could ever hope for, and to my wise and winsome publisher, Maureen R. Michelson, whose intuition and expertise kept me on track. Many thanks to Maureen, Tracy Smith, Nancy Doerrfeld-Smith, and Jenny Beranek at NewSage Press for their extraordinary ability to turn a manuscript into a readable work of art.

I am eternally grateful to John Robbins for writing *Diet for a New America*, an empowering gift that transformed my life into one filled with greater awareness, compassion, and purpose.

My deepest appreciation and affection go to Michael Panarese for being present in so many ways. He is the sun in my sky.

CONTENTS

FOREWORD   *ix*

INTRODUCTION
WHY VEGETARIAN?   *xi*

CHAPTER ONE
GETTING STARTED: SO, NOW WHAT DO I EAT?   1

CHAPTER TWO
DAIRY SUBSTITUTES: *MOOVE* OVER MILK!   9

CHAPTER THREE
SOUPS AND CANNED FOODS: SOUPER SIMPLE MEALS   25

CHAPTER FOUR
TRAVELING FARE AND SAVORY SNACKS   35

CHAPTER FIVE
BURGERS AND DOGS AND MEAT ANALOGUES   43

CHAPTER SIX
DRESSINGS, DIPS, SAUCES, AND SPREADS TO RELISH   57

CHAPTER SEVEN
FROZEN MEALS: CHILLING SURPRISES   73

CHAPTER EIGHT
**FUN FOODS FOR PARTIES, HOLIDAYS,
AND SPECIAL OCCASIONS**   85

CHAPTER NINE
DESSERTS: ICE DREAMS AND BEYOND   89

CHAPTER TEN
COFFEE SUBSTITUTES: KICKING CAFFEINE   105

CHAPTER ELEVEN
SUGAR SAVVY: THE SCOOP ON SWEETENERS   111

CHAPTER TWELVE
THE PET DEPARTMENT: FLUFFY AND FIDO GO VEGGIE!   123

NETWORKING RESOURCES   135

VEGETARIAN RESOURCES ON THE INTERNET   137

GLOSSARY   142

SUGGESTED READING   148

INDEX OF SUPPLIERS   150

FOOD INDEX   164

ABOUT THE AUTHOR   166

Foreword

We are all rethinking our diets. We aim to slim down, lower our cholesterol or our blood pressure levels, or reduce the risk of cancer and heart disease, or bring down our blood pressure. Some of us just want to live longer. Or it may be that the recognition of environmental or animal rights issues motivates us to dump out the drumsticks and ham. But, then comes the question: So, now what do I eat?

As we wander down unfamiliar aisles at the grocery store and read strange ingredients in recipe lists, we ask ourselves if we really have time for healthy eating. We are torn between the convenience of greasy fast foods and the daunting prospect of relearning how to cook and how to eat, wondering if we'll ever be on terra firma again.

It gets even more complicated when you enter a health food store. Twenty years ago, health food stores were dusty, cramped places, staffed by folks in tie-died shirts who knew all twelve products on their shelves.

No more. Health food stores are now huge supermarkets with shelves overflowing with foods we once only dreamt of: Hot dogs, Canadian bacon, and burgers that taste exactly like the real thing, but with no cholesterol or animal fat at all; and milk that comes from rice or soy, rather than from a cow, giving the consumer dozens of flavors ready to splash on cereal, with no animal proteins or lactose.

The Complete Guide to Vegetarian Convenience Foods presents a banquet of choices for those who are looking for convenience without sacrificing taste. Gail Davis walks down the grocery aisle with you and shows you the best choices to suit your needs. She knows the challenges of changing your personal menu, having first revamped her own diet years ago and having worked ever since to help others repair theirs. She shares her intimate knowledge of how to make sense of healthy eating and how to avoid its pitfalls.

The Complete Guide to Vegetarian Convenience Foods is a handy reference companion that should be on your kitchen counter next to your grocery list and in your glove compartment as you head to the store. It will save you hours of time shopping and will let you skip embarrassing purchases when you're shopping for others. It lets you make the change to healthier fare quickly and with confidence.

As you look over the wealth of practical material presented here, let me add four quick tips:

• Focus on exploration, not deprivation. For now, at least, you are experimenting, trying new tastes, new products, and maybe a new store or two. There will be many delights and probably an occasional dud. That's okay. It's what experimenting is all about.

• Transition foods can really help. Foods that look and taste like meat but that are actually vegetarian can lure even the most dyed-in-the-wool omnivore to a healthier diet.

• A complete break is much easier. Just as smokers have a harder time if they have an occasional cigarette, it is harder to leave fatty foods behind if every once in awhile you tease your taste buds with Kentucky Fried Chicken.

• Focus on the short term. Throw out the animal products and added oils, but do it only for three weeks. This kind of short-term test is much easier than the daunting prospect of a permanent change. After three weeks, you will likely find that you have lost weight, your blood pressure and cholesterol will probably have dropped, and your energy level will have improved noticeably. If you like the way you feel, stick with it.

The wisdom that Gail Davis has packed into these pages will make the transition to healthier eating a joy.

Neal D. Barnard, M.D.
President
Physicians Committee for Responsible Medicine

Introduction

WHY VEGETARIAN?

The most dangerous weapon in the arsenal of the
Homo sapiens is the table fork.
— Howard Lyman

I did not have the good sense to be born into a vegetarian family. The truth is, I had no way of even recognizing a vegetable unless it came out of a can. I grew up in New York City, under the guidance of two extremely doting, carnivorous parents. My father worked long hours and my mother was a homemaker whose responsibilities included grocery shopping and preparing our family's meals. But, my mother hated to cook, and that turned out to be fortunate for us all because she wasn't very good at it, either. So, she saw to it that we ate out often, at least two or three times per week, an awful lot in those days. We'd frequently go to the neighborhood diner where I'd usually gorge on a bacon cheeseburger with French fries, onion rings, and a Coke. Then I'd top it all off with apple crumb cake à la mode, a Napoleon, or something equally sweet and gooey. I remember these occasions fondly, because they were a welcome retreat from my mother's disastrous attempts at preparing chopped steak or meatballs and spaghetti (made with butter and ketchup).

Breakfast was not exactly a nutritional haven, either. For my mom it consisted of coffee and a cigarette. For me, it was not much better; a Twinkie or Hostess Fruit Pie and second-hand smoke.

As I detested the taste of most luncheon meats, my mother usually packed the same thing for lunch every day: cream cheese and jelly sandwiches on white bread with chocolate pudding for dessert. Could this diet have been the reason I was an overweight, lethargic, and chronically constipated child?

This story may sound all too familiar if you grew up in the late fifties or early sixties; a time when most Americans were in total darkness about nutrition and health. But we can't blame our parents for their nutritional ignorance when the majority of family physicians knew even less.

Today however, the overwhelming evidence in favor of a plant-based diet cannot be overlooked or ignored. Interest in vegetarianism is rising sharply as people continue to learn more about the personal and global implications of their dietary choices. An estimated 15 million Americans consider themselves vegetarian, and the number grows steadily by as much as a million each year.

After a Gallup poll showed that 20 percent of adults are likely to look for a restaurant that serves vegetarian items, the National Restaurant Association advised its members to feature a few vegetarian main-dish items on their menus. Even Disney's Magic Kingdom has caught on to this trend. Veggie burgers are now being sold at Disneyland and Walt Disney World amusement parks. In fact, demand for the meatless patties has been continually rising since first being introduced in 1994.

Why do people decide to become vegetarian? The answers vary widely. Some cite the atrocities that animals must endure even before they are slaughtered. Many people who love animals realize the incongruence of calling some animals pets, and others dinner. There are those who are concerned about the harmful environmental effects of a meat-based diet, while many others realize the impact that their food choices have upon world hunger. Millions are starving in third world countries while their grain is exported to fatten cattle to feed people in affluent nations. Still others eliminate meat from their diets simply because it is healthier. Heart disease, breast, prostate, and colon cancer, diabetes, stroke, osteoporosis and many other life-threatening illnesses are directly linked to meat-based diets.

Some people change their eating habits overnight, while others make the transition to a more wholesome diet gradually. Personally, there was not a moment's hesitation for me. After reading John Robbins' *Diet for a New America*, never did I once look back. Giving up animal-based foods had nothing to do with deprivation as far as I was concerned, and that's an important point. I love to eat and being vegetarian has opened a whole new world of delightful options for my tastebuds to explore.

Whatever reasons you may have for choosing a vegetarian diet, this book is for you. Even if you still eat chicken or fish, chances are you know someone who is a vegetarian. Perhaps it's your teenager who arrives home from college with the unexpected news that she no longer eats meat, eggs, or dairy, leaving you to wonder what on earth you will feed her. (Warning: many vegetarian teens have been known to convert a parent or two.) Or maybe you've invited the boss over for dinner, and in the midst of preparing your famous Chicken Kiev, you receive an unexpected phone call from him. He just wants to let you know that he is a strict vegetarian. Great, how do you make Kiev without chicken?

This book will make it simple for anyone to prepare and enjoy delicious plant-based meals in only a few minutes. There are no new complicated recipes to decipher, or expensive gadgets to buy. Within these pages you will learn about exciting new vegetarian foods with tastes and textures that are amazingly similar to the animal products they imitate but without the animal protein or cholesterol. Imagine meatless sausage, dairyless cheese, and fishless tuna that taste incredible and even smell much like their animal-based counterparts. Discover a wide variety of burgers, burritos, and beverages made from nuts, grains, and tofu. Prepare your palate for tantalizing dishes made from exotic-sounding ingredients like tempeh, seitan, and amazake.

The best part of all, is that thousands of healthful foods like these are readily available at your local natural foods store and many are even showing up on supermarket shelves. It's easier than you think. You just need to know what to look for. So relax, turn the page, and take a journey with me into the exciting world of vegetarian convenience foods!

CHAPTER 1

Getting Started:
So, Now What
Do I Eat?

The gods created certain kinds of beings to replenish our bodies...they are the trees and the plants and the seeds...
— Plato

A diet comprised entirely of organic whole fruits, vegetables, nuts, seeds, legumes, and grains is the ideal sustenance for humans. But, as we navigate through our hectic modern lives we often seek to find nourishment in foods that are conveniently prepackaged and ready to eat. The delicious, vegetarian food items listed in this book will fulfill that need. However, I cannot stress strongly enough how important it is that you include as many fresh, whole, organic fruits and vegetables in your diet as possible. This is easily accomplished by tossing a large, colorful vegetable salad and serving it along with each meal, and by eating fresh, whole fruits throughout the day. You might choose melon as an appetizer, berries for dessert, and an orange, apple, banana, or peach as a snack.

Although there is no human requirement for any foods of animal origin, we have been influenced since childhood to think otherwise. Through clever advertising campaigns directed at both children and adults, the meat, egg, and dairy industries have us convinced that without their products, we would all hover on the brink of malnutrition.

From an early age, children are taught that without these

foods, they will not grow big and strong. As adults, we continue clinging to this erroneous idea and unwittingly pass this belief on to our own children. Meanwhile, the media blitz continues, reinforcing the already ingrained nutritional lunacy. It is evidenced by the most frequently asked question of vegetarians: "But, *where* do you get your protein?"

That question is easily answered, but first, let's define vegetarian. A vegetarian diet excludes all meat products, such as beef, poultry, lamb, pork, and seafood. A person who eats chicken is *not* a vegetarian. (Although many people who eat poultry and fish may think of themselves as vegetarian.) A person consuming no animal flesh, but eating eggs and dairy, is referred to as a lacto-ovo vegetarian.

A strict vegetarian, or dietary vegan (pronounced vee-gun) has eliminated all products of animal origin from his or her diet including dairy, eggs, gelatin, and even honey. The foods listed in this book are predominantly vegan. The only two exceptions are foods containing honey (identified by an ❶ symbol) and products containing casein (identified by a ❸ symbol). Casein or caseinate refers to a milk protein present in many otherwise dairy-free foods. Manufacturers claim that using casein improves the taste, consistency, melting, and stretching properties of soy cheese and other products.

Protein

Vegetarians and vegans alike easily meet their protein requirement by eating a varied diet of vegetables, grains, and legumes. Consuming a variety of these foods sufficient to meet your caloric needs ensures that you will get enough protein in your diet. On the other hand, people who subsist on the Standard American Diet typically consume twice the amount of protein required by the human body. In case you are thinking that you cannot consume too much protein, bear in mind that excessive protein intake leads to osteoporosis and overworks the kidneys, liver, and digestive system.

Calcium

Many people wonder how vegans obtain their calcium. Although we have been led to believe that dairy products are the best source of this essential mineral, many plant foods provide the necessary calcium we need (without depleting it from our bodies at the same time). Excessive protein intake depletes the body of calcium, so that when you drink a glass of milk, you later excrete the calcium in your urine. Contrary to popular belief, osteoporosis (wasting away of the bone tissue), is not a disease of calcium deficiency, but rather of calcium depletion.

Dark, leafy, green vegetables are an excellent source of calcium. These include kale, collard greens, and spinach. Broccoli is also high in calcium as are soybeans, tofu, (particularly tofu made with calcium sulfate), tempeh, sesame seeds, figs, sea vegetables, molasses, and almonds. Many soy and rice milks are also fortified with calcium. One simple way to get calcium into your diet is to substitute dark leafy greens for lettuce (which has negligible nutritional value). Try using collard or other greens on a burger or sandwich, in salads, and shredded and sprinkled over cooked grains or pasta dishes. It's colorful, nutritious, and delicious.

Iron

Dark leafy greens also provide us with another essential nutrient, iron. Other iron-rich foods include dried beans, blackstrap molasses, and dried fruits such as raisins and figs.

Vitamins

A varied diet of vegetables, fruits, legumes, and grains contains bountiful quantities of vitamin A (in the form of beta-carotene), vitamin C, and vitamin E. Exposure to sunlight ensures your body will manufacture all the vitamin D it requires.

The Recommended Dietary Allowance for vitamin B12 is only 2 micrograms per day. However, it can be a bit tricky to obtain on a vegan diet. B12, necessary for healthy nerves and blood, is produced by bacteria naturally present in soil and water. Industrial agricultural practices have resulted in chemical pollution that has killed off many of these microorganisms. Eating vegetables freshly pulled from the ground and drinking water alone, will no longer guarantee us a sufficient supply of B12. Because B12 is also present in the intestines of animals, carnivores and lacto-ovo vegetarians derive sufficient quantities of B12 from their diets. However, it is not necessary to include animal products in your diet to get B12. Reliable vegan sources of B12 include fortified breakfast cereals, soy milks, and rice beverages. Red Star Nutritional Yeast, which adds an appealing cheese-like flavor to foods, is also a great source of B12. Another way to ensure you are getting this essential vitamin, is by taking a multi-vitamin or vitamin B12 supplements.

Cholesterol and Fat

All of the foods listed in this book are completely cholesterol-free. Many products are fat-free or low-fat making these foods sound choices for a heart-healthy diet. Foods that are fat-free are identified by the ♥ symbol. Many recent scientific studies show that no more than 15 percent of our daily calories should come from fat and all health experts agree that the amount of fat consumed by the average American should be drastically reduced.

There are many completely vegetarian foods that are excluded from this book because they contain hydrogenated or partially hydrogenated oils (otherwise known as "trans-fatty acids"). Unlike other vegetable oils, these oils are high in saturated fat. When you eat foods containing artery-clogging hydrogenated oils, your body responds by producing cholesterol. You may as well eat lard!

Hydrogenated oils are liquid oils that have been chemically altered to be solid at room temperature. Manufacturers use them because they are cheap, have a long shelf life, and add a smooth texture to foods. Products containing any of these oils should be avoided. Also, beware of products containing soy margarine. They usually contain hydrogenated soybean oil, although it may not be listed on the product label as such.

So, What's for Breakfast?

You will find that when you are transitioning to a vegetarian diet, breakfast is the most effortless meal of the day. Without even realizing it, you are probably already eating predominantly vegetarian fare for breakfast.

The best breakfasts include fruit. You can quickly blend a fresh fruit smoothie, (see the recipe on page 15) or top any cold cereal with sliced bananas, raisins, or berries, and sprinkle hot cereals with any one of the myriad dried fruit available like dates, currants, cranberries, or cherries. There is an abundant assortment of packaged multi-grain cereals to choose from, over which you can pour one of the many dairy-free alternatives to cow's milk listed in Chapter Two. Hot cereal choices include oatmeal, farina, cream of wheat, and multi-grain varieties made from various combinations of rye, barley, buckwheat, and rice. Granola is another delicious option; just watch out for the fat content. Choose low-fat varieties when you shop for granola.

Two wonderful breakfast standbys are hearty whole grain toast, and bagels topped with a dollop of fruit-only preserves (see pages 69-72), a schmear of cream cheese alternative (see page 23), or Spectrum Spread (see page 72). Bagels now come in so many creative varieties, it's hard to choose. I usually enjoy my bagels plain and untoasted. After all, what do you really need to add to a banana walnut bagel? It's a complete eating experience all by itself! Once only found in places like New York and Chicago, almost every town in America now boasts at least one bagel bakery. Just stay away from the egg bagels and if you're not sure of the ingredients, ask the bagel baker.

If you like muffins, which are typically loaded with cholesterol, sugar, and fat, you're in luck. Muscle Muffins™ in Bellevue, Washington will ship their fresh, nutritious muffin mixes right to your door. They come in four delicious varieties: Cornmeal Soynut, Date-Pumpkin, Walnut-Raisin, and Carob Brownie. Each bag makes twelve, plump 5 oz. muffins. All you do is grind the flax seeds (a coffee grinder works best), add soy or rice milk, and bake!

These delightful muffins are sweetened with fructose, packed with fiber, high in protein, and have no added fat or oil.

For the more adventurous, there are many wonderful recipes for vegan muffins, scrambled tofu, pancakes, waffles, and even French toast. For those of you ready to take the next step in your vegetarian evolution and begin exploring fun and exciting recipe ideas, I highly recommend *The Peaceful Palate* by Jennifer Raymond. Within its pages you will find a delightful collection of delicious, low-fat, and simple-to-prepare vegan recipes.

Product Labels

Always read product labels! I cannot overstress this point. In addition to checking the nutritional value of the item, be sure to read the listed ingredients. There are many foods excluded from this book because they contain products derived from animals or hydrogenated oils. You may go shopping and discover that I have not listed a particular flavor or variety in a given product line. Careful inspection of the label may reveal the inclusion of an objectionable ingredient in that flavor or variety. Ingredients to watch out for in otherwise healthy-sounding vegetarian food items include: whey, butter, milk solids, hydrogenated or partially hydrogenated oil, soy margarine, (usually contains hydrogenated soybean oil), gelatin, anchovies, and egg whites (which may also be listed as "albumin").

Where Do I Buy It?

If you can't find it, ask for it! Most of the products you will learn about in this book will be readily available at your local natural foods store. Supermarkets are beginning to stock natural food items in an effort to recover some of the consumer dollars lost to the growing number of health food stores. A few food companies that traditionally catered to traditional American dietary tastes, have expanded their product lines to include healthy, vegetarian alternatives. If you cannot find a particular item, seek out the store manager or buyer for that item. More often than not, the store will try to accommodate special requests to bring in an item. The best way to get a product you want into a store, is simply to ask for it.

In some cases, a store may not be able to get a special request item in house. Their distributors may not carry the product, or in the case of some natural food stores, their policy may restrict them from stocking a particular item.

Above each product entry in this book, you will find the name of the company that manufactures, imports, or distributes the product. At the back of the book is a supplier's index that lists the name, address, and phone number of each company. You are encouraged to contact these suppliers directly if you are unable to purchase a product at your local store. Manufacturers want to know if their products are not readily available to the customers who want them. They may even be able to direct you to a store in your area that carries the item you are looking for. Also, many suppliers provide retail mail order service and will ship products right to your front door. These companies are highlighted with an asterisk in the index.

If you are lucky enough to live within driving distance of a Trader Joe's market, I strongly urge you to discover this marvel of modern discount food shopping. Not only will you find many of the more popular items listed in this book at drastically reduced prices, but TJ's has an abundance of prepared vegetarian convenience foods manufactured under its own private label, including delicious fresh fruit smoothies and ethnic entrées.

Share Your Food Finds!

Exciting, new, completely vegetarian convenience foods are constantly being developed and introduced into the market. The natural foods industry is growing so rapidly that you will likely discover some of these products on your own. If you find a new item not mentioned in this book, and would like to share your discovery with others, please write and tell me about it. I'll be happy to include your food finds in subsequent editions of *The Complete Guide to Vegetarian Convenience Foods*. Please send product information to: Gail Davis, P.O. Box 2101, Corrales, New Mexico 87048 or e-mail me at: VegieGail@aol.com.

The Difference Your Food Choices Make

Few of us realize the awesome power of our dietary choices. Just by consciously deciding to center our diets around plant-based foods we can drastically reduce our risk of heart disease, stroke, diabetes, osteoporosis, and breast, prostate, and colon cancers. We can help put an end to the extraordinary human suffering caused by hunger and malnutrition. We can effectively stop the senseless destruction of our world's rainforests that produce 80 percent of the Earth's oxygen. We can significantly address our environmental concerns by reducing the toxic pollution of our air, soil, and water.

Did you know that animal agriculture accounts for more pollution of our country's waters than all other sources combined? We can cut down on the thoughtless waste of these precious natural resources, which are not limitless. We can teach our children to become more loving and compassionate human beings by ceasing to raise them on the suffering of sentient creatures. Imagine all of the power is just sitting at the center of our plates!

Key to Symbols

For the following chapters I have created a guide to help you navigate through the listings. The "Key to Symbols" will be indicated at the beginning of each chapter.

❤ Fat Free
✍ Author's Favorite
✤ Kid's Pick
Ⓒ Contains casein or caseinate
Ⓗ Contains honey

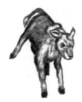

CHAPTER 2

Dairy Substitutes: *Moove* Over Milk!

There is no biological need for milk.
— Suzanne Havala, M.S., R.D.
American Dietetic Association's
Position Paper on Vegetarian Diets

Milk

Soy, rice, almond, and oat beverages are all delicious alternatives to cow's milk. They come in several flavors, with fat-free and enriched versions. Most are packaged in aseptic cartons (known as Tetra Paks®), and have a shelf life of about one year. Once opened, they require refrigeration. Soy milks will then last about a week, while rice and almond beverages will last up to ten days. Newer to the market are powdered versions of these beverages. They're a real lifesaver when traveling, since they come in small, easy-to-carry packages and you can mix only as much as you need.

Soy milks are thick and creamy and have a rather strong, distinctive taste. They are wonderful for making exotic coffee drinks, shakes, and for use in all types of recipes. Chocolate soy milk is absolutely delicious and a favorite among kids.

Rice milk has a lighter consistency much like 2 percent dairy milk and is generally lower in fat. Vanilla rice milk is delicious in coffee drinks, poured over cereal, or enjoyed straight out of the carton.

Key to Symbols:	♥ Fat Free ✍ Author's Favorite ✿ Kid's Pick
	© Contains casein or caseinate ℍ Contains honey

Almond milk and oat milk each boast a unique flavor. They are completely versatile and tasty as beverages, poured over cereal, or added to recipes.

Soy Milk

EDEN FOODS, INC.

EdenSoy®
Rich, creamy taste in Original, Vanilla, or Carob.

EdenSoy® Extra
Fortified with antioxidents, vitamins, and minerals in Original and Vanilla.

FIRST LIGHT FOODS

Soy-Um™
Rich, creamy taste in Original, Vanilla, or Chocolate ❀ ✍.

FULLER LIFE, INC.

Hearty Life™ Better Than Milk™ ✍.
Real dairy taste in the Original flavor.

THE HAIN FOOD GROUP, INC.

Soy Supreme™
Original and Vanilla.

HEALTH VALLEY FOODS

Fat-Free Soy Moo ♥
Great tasting; flavored with vanilla.

IMAGINE FOODS, INC.

Soy Dream®
From the makers of Rice Dream®. Extremely rich, refreshing taste. Original ✍ and Vanilla ✍ are ideal for cooking and baking. Also comes in Carob flavor.

Soy Dream® Enriched 🖎
Great tasting and fortified with calcium and vitamins A, D, E,
and B12. Original, Vanilla, and Chocolate ✿.

INTERNATIONAL PROSOYA CORP.

So Nice™ Soymilk 🖎
So much great taste in fresh (refrigerated) or Tetra Pak®
cartons. You'll be amazed at how much like dairy milk the
Original flavor tastes! If you enjoy the taste of moo-milk,
this product was made just for you. Natural, Vanilla,
Original, and Chocolate ✿.

INTERNOVA INC.

Nutrisoy
Great tasting soy beverage enriched with calcium
and vitamins A, B2, and D. Original and Vanilla 🖎.

PACIFIC FOODS OF OREGON, INC.

Pacific Original Soymilk
Unsweetened Original flavor.

Pacific Select Soy Drink
Low fat, low sodium beverage for price conscious
shoppers in Plain or Vanilla.

Pacific Fat Free Soy Drink ❤
Plain and Vanilla.

QUICK TIP: PERK UP HOT BEVERAGES!

Instead of adding cream and sugar to coffee, (refer to Chapter
Ten for great coffee substitutes) or milk and honey to tea, stir
in vanilla soy milk. It's a sweet and delicious alternative to
traditional hot beverage additives. It's perfect for making latté
and cappuccino drinks, too.

Pacific Enriched Soy Drink
Enriched with calcium, riboflavin, and vitamins A and D.
In Plain, Vanilla, and Cocoa.

Pacific Ultra Soy Drink
Fortified with vitamins and minerals, as well as L. Acidophilus
and L. Bifidus to aid in digestion. Plain and Vanilla.

VITASOY, INC.

Vitasoy®
Creamy Original, Vanilla Delite, Carob Supreme,
and Rich Cocoa ❀.

Vitasoy® Enriched
With added calcium, riboflavin, zinc, and vitamins A, D,
and B12. Original and Vanilla.

Vitasoy® Light
Only 1% fat in Original, Vanilla, and Cocoa.

WESTBRAE NATURAL FOODS

Westsoy® Organic
33% more protein than milk. In Original and Unsweetened.

Westsoy® Plus
Fortified with calcium, vitamins A and D, and riboflavin.
Plain, Vanilla, and Cocoa ❀.

Westsoy® Lite
Only 1% fat in Plain, Vanilla, or Cocoa.

Westsoy® Non Fat ❤
Plain and Vanilla.

Westsoy® Soy Drink
Made with malted cereal extract containing barley; has less
sugar, but the same great taste as other Westsoy milks.
Available in Plain and Vanilla.

Westsoy® Concentrate
Economical, makes 2 quarts. Plain and Vanilla.

Westsoy® Original Malteds
These refreshing dessert beverages in handy single-serving packages don't really taste like malteds, but they're rich and satisfying. Vanilla, Cocoa-Mint, Almond, Java, and Carob.

Westsoy® Lite Malteds
Half the fat and ⅓ fewer calories. Vanilla Royale, Cocoa-Mint, Carob, Almond, and Creamy Banana.

Westsoy® VigorAid Nutritional Drink™
Much more than a soy beverage, VigorAid is packed with 25 vitamins, minerals and phytonutrients. In single-serving boxes. French Vanilla, Creamy Chocolate, and Chocolate Mocha.

WHITE WAVE, INC.

Silk™
Delicious tasting, vanilla flavored soy milk. Found fresh in your grocer's dairy case.

Chocolate Silk ❀
Fresh tasting chocolaty flavor.

Organic Silk™

Rice Milk

AMERICAN NATURAL SNACKS

Harmony Farms™ Fat-Free Rice Drink ❤
Original and Vanilla.

FIRST LIGHT FOODS

Rice-Um™
Original and Vanilla.

THE HAIN FOOD GROUP, INC.

Rice Supreme™
Original and Cinnamon.

IMAGINE FOODS, INC.

Rice Dream®
The original light, refreshing rice beverage. Original, Vanilla ✍, Carob, or Chocolate ✿.

Rice Dream® Enriched
Fortified with calcium and vitamins A and D. Original, Vanilla ✍, and Chocolate ✿.

PACIFIC FOODS OF OREGON, INC.

Pacific Low Fat Rice Drink
Enriched with vitamins A and D, calcium, L. Acidophilus and L. Bifidus. Plain, Vanilla, and Cocoa.

Pacific Fat Free Rice Drink ❤
Fortified, but without any fat. Plain, Vanilla, and Cocoa.

WESTBRAE NATURAL FOODS

Westsoy® Rice Drink
Plain and Vanilla.

Westsoy® Rice Drink Concentrate
Economical, makes 2 quarts in Plain and Vanilla.

WHITE WAVE, INC.

Rice Silk™
Great fresh taste in the grocer's dairy case (refrigerated).

Almond Milk

BLUE DIAMOND GROWERS

Blue Diamond® Breeze™
Calcium enriched with vitamins A and D. No added oils.
In Original, Vanilla, and Chocolate ❀ ✍.

PACIFIC FOODS OF OREGON, INC.

Naturally Almond
Made from real almonds, without added oils. Naturally great
tasting. Original and Vanilla ❀ ✍ flavors.

Oat Milk

PACIFIC FOODS OF OREGON, INC.

Naturally Oat
Great oaty taste without added oils. Original and Vanilla.

WESTBRAE NATURAL FOODS

Oat Plus™
Wonderful oaty flavor with added vitamins A, D,
and riboflavin. Original and Vanilla.

> **QUICK TIP: BREAKFAST SMOOTHIE OF CHAMPIONS**
> Combine one cup of your favorite "milk" beverage with one
> ripe banana, ½ cup frozen strawberries, and 1 teaspoon
> natural sweetener in a blender. Mix on high speed for a
> sensational morning eye-opener.

Multi Grain Beverages

EDEN FOODS, INC.

EdenBlend® Rice & Soy Beverage
Blended rice and soy creates a delicate balance of flavors.

GALAXY FOODS CO.

Galaxy Foods® Veggie Milk™
A nutritious blend of organic soy, rice, and oats fortified with vitamins and minerals. Available in either shelf stable Tetra Pak® cartons or fresh in your supermarket's dairy case.

PACIFIC FOODS OF OREGON, INC.

Multi Grain Non Dairy Beverage
A satisfying beverage with a nutritious balance of essential amino acids. Made from a unique blend of triticale, barley, oats, soy beans, brown rice, and amaranth.

Naturally Complete™ Complete Liquid Nutrition
A unique blend of whole grains and organic soy-beans packing a powerful punch of phytonutrients, 26 vitamins and minerals, and 9 grams of high quality protein. In Vanilla and Chocolate flavors.

Potato-Based Non-Dairy Beverage

A & A AMAZING FOODS, INC.

Vance's DariFree™ (H) ❤
Made from potato extracts, this beverage tastes very much like cow's milk and contains just as much calcium, too.

Powdered Non Dairy Beverages

A & A AMAZING FOODS, INC.

Vance's DariFree™ (H) ❤
Potato-based mix free of rice, soy, corn, and oils.

DEVANSOY FARMS, INC.

Solait
Soy-based beverage mix in Plain, Vanilla, and Chocolate.

ENER-G FOODS, INC.

EnerG® Non-Dairy Beverages
Lacto-Free is a soy-based beverage mix. NutQuik is an almond-based beverage and baking mix. PureSoyQuik is made from toasted soy flour. All are free of preservatives, sugar, or artificial flavoring and come with a variety of tasty sounding recipes printed on the box.

EQUINOX INTERNATIONAL

Equi-Milk ❤
Refreshing taste, formulated with potato extracts, fructose sweetened, and supplemented with vitamins and minerals.

FULLER LIFE, INC.

Hearty Life™ Better Than Milk™ Soy
Tofu-based drink mix in Original, Light, Vanilla ⊙, Carob, and Chocolate.

Hearty Life™ Better Than Milk™ Rice ❤
Original and Vanilla flavors.

LUMEN FOODS

Heaven on Earth Fat Free Milk Replacer ❤
Tofu drink mix in Original and Carob.

MODERN PRODUCTS, INC.

Riceness® ❤
Original, Vanilla, or Chocolate.

Soyness®
Original, Vanilla, or Chocolate

Non-Dairy Creamer

WESTBRAE NATURAL FOODS

Westsoy® Lite Non Dairy Creamer
50% less fat and 50% fewer calories than half and half.
Great in coffee drinks, poured over fruit, and with cereal.

Amazake

Amazake is a thick, rich, highly energizing beverage. It is made by mixing organic brown rice with koji (a rice culture). Fresh, cold amazake tastes like a delicious dairy-free milk shake. Use it as a base for desserts, puddings, sauces, salad dressings, and smoothies. Amazake is naturally sweet (there's no added sugar) and easily digestible. Find fresh amazake in the refrigerated section of your natural food store.

GRAINAISSANCE, INC.

Grainaissance Amazake
This beverage is so satisfying and delicious, it should come with a warning label that says, "Caution: highly addictive." Original ❤, Hazelnut, Almond Shake ✍, Cocoa-Almond ❀ ✍, Sesame, Apricot ❤, Vanilla-Pecan ✍, Mocha-Java, Banana Smoothie ❤ ❀, Rice Nog ✍ (a super holiday beverage) and Coffee (made with real coffee and cocoa).

Gimme Green SuperShake ✍
A great tasting amazake beverage loaded with natural vitamins, minerals, and antioxidents from a combination of green foods. This shake has a flavorful blend of almonds and bananas.

QUICK TIP: FROZEN TREAT FOR BIG and LITTLE KIDS
Fill a popsicle maker with any flavor of amazake. Freeze to enjoy a great refreshment on a hot summer day!

Smoothies and Shakes

BLUE SKY NATURAL FOODS

Sky® Shake
Great tasting shake in a can! Soy-based, low fat, and high protein beverage. Chocolate Supreme, Vanilla Maple, and Marvelous Mocha (contains caffeine).

GOLDEN VALLEY FOODS

Advantage\10™ Fruit Smoothies ✍
A delicious and satisfying blend of soy milk, fruit, and grains with 10% or less of calories from fat. Raspberry, Strawberry, and Strawberry-Banana flavor in individual serving packages.

Cheese

Many transitioning vegetarians are unaware that most dairy cheese substitutes contain casein or caseinate, a protein derived from cow's milk. Manufacturers say that they add casein to soy and many otherwise dairyless cheeses to make the product stretch and melt when heated. Although foods containing casein are free of lactose and cholesterol, they cannot be considered completely plant-based because casein is an animal product. The **Ⓒ** symbol indicates that the product listed contains casein or caseinate.

AMERICAN NATURAL SNACKS

Soya Kaas® Ⓒ
Mozzarella, Monterey Jack, Garlic & Herb, Mild American Cheddar, and Jalapeño Mexi-Kaas.

Soya Kaas® Fat Free Ⓒ ❤
Cheddar, Jalapeño, and Mozzarella.

Soya Kaas® Grated Soy Cheese Ⓒ
Parmesan flavor.

SoyaKaas® Slices ©
American Cheddar or White American.

Vegie Kaas®
Casein-free spreads in Cheddar and Smoked Cheddar flavors.

CEMAC FOODS CORP.

Nu Tofu® Soy Cheese Alternative ©
Mozzarella, Monterey Jack, Cheddar, and Jalapeño Jack.

Nu Tofu® Fat-Free Cheeses © ❤
Mozzarella, Cheddar, Monterey Jack, and Jalapeño Jack.

NuTofu® Low Sodium Cheese Alternative ©
Mozzarella and Cheddar flavors.

The following Galaxy Foods cheeses are conveniently located in your supermarket's dairy case.

GALAXY FOODS CO.

Galaxy Foods® Tofu Slices
Original, Italian Garlic Herb, Savory, and Hickory Smoked ✍

Galaxy Foods® Veggie Slices™ ©
Provolone, Mozzarella, American, Cheddar, Swiss, Pepperjack, Mediterranean Style Bleu, Mediterranean Style Feta, and Fat Free American ❤

Galaxy Foods® Veggie Chunk ©
Cheddar and Mozzarella flavors.

Galaxy Foods® Veggie Topping ©
Grated cheese alternative in Garlic Herb and Parmesan flavors.

P.J. LISAC & ASSOCIATES, INC.

Lisanatti™ Brand Soy-Sation® © and Soy-Sation Lite ©
Excellent taste and texture. Mozzarella, Jalapeño Jack, Cheddar, and Garlic & Herb.

Lisanatti™ Almond Cheeze ☉
Mozzarella, Pepper Jack, Cheddar, and Garlic & Herb.

RELLA GOOD CHEESE CO.

TofuRella and TofuRella Slices™ ☉
Made with tofu in five flavors: Cheddar, Mozzarella,
Jalapeño Jack, Monterey Jack, and Garlic & Herb.

HempRella™ ☉
Jamaica Jack flavor made from hemp nectar.

Zero-fatRella™ ☉ ♥
Tofu based in Cheddar, Mozzarella, and Jalapeño Jack.

AlmondRella™ ☉
Made from almond milk: Cheddar, Garlic-Herb,
and Mozzarella.

VeganRella™
Made from organic brown rice milk, it's firm when cold,
melts when heated, and is casein-free. In Cheddar and
Mozzarella varieties.

RiceRella and RiceRella Slices™ ☉
In Cheddar, Mozzarella, and Hickory Smoked flavors.

Soyco Foods makes several different lines of cheese alternatives.
Soy Nutritious Lite & Less™ cheeses are soy based. The Rice,
Almond, and Oat lines are totally soy free. Soymage™ cheeses are
100% vegan and casein-free.

Grated Cheese

SOYCO FOODS

Lite & Less™ ☉
Parmesan flavor.

Rice™ Parmesan ☉

Soymage™ Parmesan ✍

Chunk Cheese and Cheese Slices

SOYCO FOODS

Almond Slices ⊙
American and Mozzarella.

Almond Low Fat Chunks ⊙
Cheddar and Mozzarella.

Lite & Less™ Veggy Singles ⊙
American ❀, Swiss, Mozzarella, Pepper Jack, and Provolone.

Lowfat Veggy Chunk ⊙
Mozzarella, Jalapeño, and Cheddar.

Fat Free Veggy Chunk ⊙ ♥
Mozzarella, Jalapeño, and Cheddar.

Oat Slices ⊙
American and Mozzarella.

Oat Low Fat Chunk ⊙
Cheddar and Mozzarella.

Rice™ Slices ⊙
American, Mozzarella, Cheddar, Pepperjack, and Swiss.

Rice™ Low Fat Chunk ⊙
Mozzarella and Cheddar.

Soymage™ SoySingles™ ♥
Mozzarella and American styles.

Soymage™ Chunk ✍
Mozzarella, Cheddar, Jalapeño, and Italian Herb.

WHITE WAVE, INC.

Soy A Melt Soy Cheeses ⊙
Jalapeño, Garlic, Herb, Cheddar, and Mozzarella.

Soy A Melt Fat Free Soy Cheeses Ⓒ ❤
Mozzarella and Cheddar.

Cream Cheese

AMERICAN NATURAL SNACKS

Soya Kaas™ Cream Cheese Ⓒ ✍
Creamy texture in Plain, Garlic & Herb, Garden Vegetable,
and Strawberry flavors.

GALAXY FOODS CO.

Galaxy Foods® Veggie Cream Cheese Ⓒ ✍
Made with organic tofu and lower in fat than traditional
cream cheese. Found in your supermarket's dairy case.

SOYCO FOODS

Rice™ Low Fat Cream Cheese Ⓒ

Soymage™ Low Fat Cream Cheese

Sour Cream

GALAXY FOODS CO.

Galaxy Foods® Veggie Sour Cream Ⓒ
Low fat alternative to sour cream made with organic tofu.
Look for it in the dairy section of your supermarket.

SOYCO FOODS

Soymage™ Sour Cream
100% dairyless and tastes great!

Rice™ Low Fat Sour Cream Ⓒ

Yogurt

INTERNATIONAL PROSOYA CORP.

So Nice™ Soy Yogurt ✍ ❀
So much delicious taste in Fieldberry, Strawberry, Black
Cherry, Raspberry, and Vanilla.

SPRINGFIELD CREAMERY

Nancy's Soy Yogurt Treats
Contain active yogurt cultures. Plain ❶, Blackberry, Blueberry,
Strawberry, Kiwi/Lime, Mango, and Vanilla.

WHITE WAVE, INC.

Dairyless Soy Yogurt
Organic Plain, Raspberry, Lemon, Strawberry, Blueberry,
Peach, Lemon-Kiwi, Banana-Strawberry, Key Lime,
Apricot-Mango, Vanilla, Orange Creme, and Cappuccino.

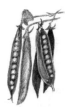

CHAPTER 3

Soups and Canned Foods: Souper Simple Meals

How good it is to be well-fed, healthy, and kind, all at the same time.
— Henry Heimlich, M.D.

Soups

Healthy, delicious, vegetarian soups are widely available in cans, cups, cartons, and convenient, slim packages. Included here are soups that are low-fat or completely fat-free and have passed my rigorous taste testing to screen out the bland and the ordinary. Many soups are hearty enough to make a complete meal by themselves (as are all of the chilis). But since you need not live by soup alone, you can toss a salad of fresh greens and raw vegetables, serve with a hunk of crusty whole-grain bread, and enjoy a wholesome, nutritious, and satisfying meal in minutes.

DR. McDOUGALL'S RIGHT FOODS, INC.

Dr. McDougall's Soups ✍
Great tasting, low fat soup in a cup. Minestrone & Pasta, Split Pea with Barley, and Tortilla Soup with Baked Chips ❀.

Key to Symbols:	♥ Fat Free ✍ Author's Favorite ❀ Kid's Pick
	Ⓒ Contains casein or caseinate **Ⓗ** Contains honey

Ramen Noodles ✍ ❀
Baked, not fried! Completely vegetarian. Chicken
and Beef flavors.

Energy Cup Instant Meals ✍
Tamale Pie with Baked Chips ❀, Pinto Beans & Rice,
Southwestern Style Pasta with Beans, Chicken Flavor,
and Mediterranean Style Rice & Pasta Pilaf.

EDWARD & SONS TRADING CO., INC.

Organic Country Bouillon Cubes
Great flavor and convenience for soups, stews, sauces,
noodles, or rice dishes. In two flavors: Harvest Vegetable
and Herb Medley.

FANTASTIC FOODS, INC.

Fantastic Foods Hearty Soup Cups
Jumpin' Black Bean, Split Pea, Cha Cha Cha Chili ✍,
Country Lentil, Couscous with Lentils, Five Bean,
and Vegetable Barley.

Fantastic Foods Couscous Cups
Black Bean Salsa, Creole Vegetable, and Sweet Corn. ✍

Fantastic Foods Only a Pinch Soup Cups
Couscous with Lentils and Spanish Rice and Beans.

Fantastic Ramen Noodles Soup Cups
Chicken Free, Vegetable Curry, Vegetable Miso,
and Vegetable Tomato.

GEETHA'S GOURMET PRODUCTS

Geetha's Gourmet Dal Lentil Soup ♥
Truly thick and hearty with the savory flavors of India.

HARVEST DIRECT, INC.

Harvest Direct® Vegetarian Broths ♥
The ultimate in convenience. Dry broth mixes are great

for soups and stocks. All five realistic tasting flavors are completely free of animal products. Just add one cup of boiling water to two teaspoons of broth. Beef, Chicken ✍, Vegetable, Ham, and Seafood flavored broths.

HEALTH VALLEY FOODS, INC.

Organic Soups ✪ ❤
These canned soups are also available in No Salt Added versions: Minestrone, Potato Leek, Lentil, Tomato, Vegetable, Black Bean, Split Pea, and Mushroom-Barley.

Fat-Free Healthy Soup In A Cup ❤
Spicy Black Bean with Couscous, Chicken Flavored Noodles with Vegetable (no chicken), Zesty Black Bean with Rice, Lentil with Couscous, and Garden Split Pea with Carrots.

Fat-Free Soup ✪ ❤
Canned soups: Vegetable Barley, Split Pea and Carrots, Country Corn & Vegetable, Black Bean & Vegetable, Lentil & Carrots, 5 Bean Vegetable, 14 Garden Vegetable, and Tomato Vegetable.

Fat-Free Carotene Soup ✪ ❤
Contains 25,000 IU of beta-carotene. Vegetable Power, Italian Plus, and Super Broccoli in cans.

IMAGINE FOODS, INC.

Imagine Natural® Garden Vegetable Soups
Scrumptious taste, low in fat, and packaged in ultra-convenient, resealable Tetra Pak® cartons. The Creamy Butternut Squash ✍ is sensational. Also: Creamy Broccoli, Zesty Gazpacho ❤, Creamy Mushroom, No-Chicken Broth, Creamy Potato Leek, Creamy Sweet Corn, Creamy Tomato, and Vegetable Broth.

NILE SPICE FOODS

Nile Spice™ Cups of Soup
Black Bean, Chili & Corn ✍, Lentil, Minestrone, Red Beans & Rice, or Split Pea.

PACIFIC FOODS OF OREGON, INC.

Chef's Classics® Instant Soups
Low-fat and flavorful soup cups. Black Bean, Minestrone, Savory Lentil and Rice ❶, Cajun Red Beans and Rice, Caribbean Black Beans and Rice, and Curried Lentils & Rice.

Pacific Organic All Natural Broths ♥
Perfect for recipes or enjoy alone. They come in convenient, resealable Tetra Pak® cartons. Vegetable Broth and Mushroom Broth varieties.

PROGRESSO QUALITY FOODS COMPANY

Progresso® Lentil Soup ✍
Tasty and hearty canned soup.

SAHARA NATURAL FOODS, INC.

Casbah® Teapot Soups ✍
These soups come in eco-friendly single-serving packets. Great for traveling or camping. You provide the cup and save money, too. Santa Fe Rice & Beans, Hearty Lentil, Chicken Noodle (all vegetarian), Sweet Corn Chowder, Garden Couscous, Vegetarian Chili, Milano Minestrone, Potato Leek, Split Pea, Black Bean, Mexicana Couscous, and Vegetarian Chicken Almondine Couscous.

SCENARIO INTERNATIONAL, INC.

The Organic Gourmet™ Soup Bases ♥
For a hearty soup, just add your favorite vegetables or use alone for a light, satisfying broth. Also make great bases for gravies. Wild Mushroom Soup 'N Stock, Vegetable Soup 'N Stock, and Vegetable Bouillon Cubes.

SEENERGY FOODS LTD.

Nature's Chef™ Premium Soups
These soups come frozen in convenient stand-up pouches. The 7 Vegetable Minestrone and Southwest Black Bean varieties are dairy-free.

SHARIANN'S ORGANICS, INC.

ShariAnn's™ Organic Gourmet Soups
Canned soups with international flair: Spicy French Green
Lentil ♥, Italian White Bean with Herb ❶, Spicy Mexican
Bean, Indian Black Bean & Rice, Great Plains Split Pea ❶ ♥,
Tomato with Roasted Garlic ❶ ♥, Tomato with Roasted Red
Bell Pepper ♥, and Vegetarian French Onion ♥ ✍.

TRADITION FOODS INC.

Tradition Naturals Ramen Noodle Soup ✍
The Fiesta Vegetable flavor is 98% fat free and delicious.

WESTBRAE NATURAL FOODS

Fat Free Soups of the World ♥
Canned Hearty Milano Minestrone, Alabama Black
Bean Gumbo, Louisiana Bean Stew, Santa Fe Vegetable,
Great Plains Savory Bean, Old World Split Pea, Rich
Mediterranean Lentil, Wellington UnBeef Barley, and
Versailles Garden Vegetable.

WILL-PAK FOODS, INC.

Taste Adventure Soups
Homemade taste in stay-fresh multiple-serving cartons. Split
Pea, Black Bean, Curry Lentil, Minestrone ❀, Navy Bean ♥,
Golden Pea, and Sweet Corn Chowder ✍.

WOODSTOCK ORGANICS

Organic All Natural Soups ❶
Wholesome goodness and 99% fat free! These frozen soups
are made with a savory blend of vegetables, herbs, and
seasonings. Vegetable Barley, Split Pea, Lentil, and Power
Lunch Vegetarian Stew.

Chili

ARROWHEAD MILLS, INC.

Arrowhead Mills® All Natural Chili ⊕
Plump organic beans in a savory chili sauce. Panhandle Vegetarian, Mild Black Bean, and Spicy Black Bean.

FANTASTIC FOODS, INC.

Chile Olé™
Black bean chili with corn in a cup.

GREENE'S FARM

Greene's Farm® Vegetarian Chili ⊕ ✍ ❀
Great tasting organically grown 3-bean chili in a can.

HEALTH VALLEY FOODS, INC.

Fat-Free Chili ⊕ ♥
Fajita Flavor, Mild Vegetarian with 3 Beans, Mild Vegetarian with Black Beans, or Spicy Vegetarian with Black Beans.

QUICK TIP: POTATO TOPPERS

Here's the perfect idea for leftover soup and chili. Store in refrigerator until ready to use. Bake some potatoes (4-8 minutes in microwave on high). Top potatoes with reheated soup or chili and serve!

No-Fat Added Chili ⊕
Also available in No Salt Added. Mild Vegetarian Chili with Lentils ♥ Spicy Vegetarian Chili with Organic Beans (only 1 gm. of fat), and Mild Vegetarian Chili with Organic Beans ♥.

HORMEL FOODS CORPORATION

Hormel® Vegetarian Chili with Beans ❤
Flavorful chili loaded with kidney beans.

Stagg® 99% Fat Free Vegetable Garden™ Chili ✍
Full of flavor four-bean chili made with a zesty variety of vegetables, herbs, and spices.

LITTLE BEAR ORGANIC FOODS

Bearitos® Low Fat Premium Chili
Original, Spicy, and Black Bean.

SHARIANN'S ORGANICS, INC.

ShariAnn's® Organic Veggie Chili ⊕
Also available: Spicy Veggie Chili.

WILL-PAK FOODS, INC.

Taste Adventure Chili
Homemade taste in stay-fresh multiple-serving cartons—just add water: Black Bean, Red Bean ❀, Lentil, and 5 Bean Chili varieties.

WOLF BRAND PRODUCTS

Wolf® Brand Chunky Vegetable Chili ✍
Tasty blend of pinto, kidney, and black beans in a savory tomato sauce.

YVES VEGGIE CUISINE INC.

Yves Veggie Chili ✍
Made with Yves Veggie Ground Round, whole red kidney beans, fresh tomatoes, red and green bell peppers, carrots, and onions, and simmered in a savory blend of herbs and spices.

Baked Beans

Serve with veggie hot dogs, as a side dish to veggie cold cut sandwiches, with barbecue tempeh, or over a bed of rice.

BUSH BROTHERS & COMPANY

Bush's Best Vegetarian Baked Beans ✍ ❤ ❀
The best vegetarian baked beans by far.

HEALTH VALLEY FOODS, INC.

Fat-Free Honey Baked Beans ⓗ ❤
Available in No Salt Added version. Contains Certified Organic Beans.

Refried Beans

A favorite of Mexican food connoisseurs. These vegetarian varieties are all made without lard.

HUNT-WESSON, INC.

Rosarita® Vegetarian Refried Beans
98% Fat Free Vegetarian, Low Fat Black Bean, No Fat Traditional ❤, No Fat Zesty Salsa ❤, and No Fat Green Chile and Lime ❤.

LITTLE BEAR ORGANIC FOODS

Bearitos® Low Fat Refried Beans
Regular Pinto, Spicy Pinto, No Salt, and Black Bean.

Bearitos Fat Free Refried Beans ❤
Regular, Green Chili, or Black Bean.

SHARIANN'S ORGANICS, INC.

ShariAnn's™ Refried Beans ❤
Black Bean, Pinto Bean, Pintos with Roasted Garlic, Black Beans with Roasted Red Jalapeño, and Pintos with Green Chili & Lime.

Rice and Beans

FANTASTIC FOODS, INC.

Fantastic Foods Rice & Bean Cups
Cajun with Red Beans and Spicy Jamaican with Black Beans.

LITTLE BEAR ORGANIC FOODS

Bearitos Beans and Rice
Cajun Style ❶, Mexican Style, and Cuban Style.

WILL-PAK FOODS, INC.

Taste Adventure Quick Cuisine
Fast dishes in handy cartons are ready in ten minutes or less. Just add hot water and simmer. For an even heartier meal, just add tofu or vegetables. Jambalaya, Bombay Curry ✍, and Santa Fe Fiesta.

QUICK TIP: SIMPLY SOUPER SALAD
Prepare Santa Fe Fiesta Quick Cuisine and allow to cool. Add 1 cup diced tomatoes, 2 tablespoons olive oil, 1 teaspoon vinegar, 1 tablespoon fresh parsley or cilantro and chill.

Macaroni and Cheese

ROAD'S END ORGANICS, INC.

Dairy-Free macaroni and chReese™ ❀
The original vegan alternative to the classic cheesy dish.
Nutritional yeast flakes give this product its chReesy flavor.
Low fat, organic ingredients, and a great source of vitamin
B12.

Dairy-Free shells and chReese™

Dairy-Free rice penne and chReese™
A new wheat-free variety.

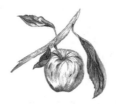

CHAPTER 4

Traveling Fare
and Savory Snacks

If it has eyes or runs away, don't eat it.
— William Keith Kellogg

Camping Foods

Camping foods are transportable meals you can take with you anywhere; they are not just for camping. You can bring them to the office, on a long airline flight or train trip, to your hotel room, on a bicycling or sailing excursion, and of course, when you go camping. These foods are lightweight and convenient. The most you will need is access to heat and water. In addition to the foods you'll find in this section, the many cup and package soups listed in Chapter Three are lightweight and convenient for traveling, as are the powdered "milks" listed in Chapter Two.

ALPINEAIRE FOODS™

Naturally good food for the outdoor gourmet. Perfect for camping and backpacking, these fully dehydrated foods are completely vegetarian and come in easy-to-carry, lightweight packages:

Key to Symbols:	♥ Fat Free ✍ Author's Favorite ❀ Kid's Pick
	☉ Contains casein or caseinate ☉ Contains honey

Alpine Minestrone Soup
Apple Almond Crisp ⓗ
Apple Sauce with Cinnamon ❤
Chili
Couscous
French Cut Green Beans Almondine
Garden Vegetables ❤
GOT'M (Good Old Trail Mix)
Granola
Hash Browns and Greens ❤
Macaroni-Vegetable ❤
Macaroni-Whole Wheat ❤
Mashed Potatoes, Instant ❤
Mountain Chili
Multi Bean Soup
Mushroom Pilaf with Vegetables ❤
Peaches, Diced ❤
Peanut Butter Pouches
Pineapple Chunks ❤
Santa Fe Black Beans and Rice
Spaghetti Marinara with Mushrooms ⓗ
Sweet Bell Pepper Combo ❤
Wild Rice Pilaf with Almonds

BACKPACKER'S PANTRY

no-cook Meals by Backpacker's Pantry
Just add boiling water to the stand-up pouches and
a delicious hot meal is ready in minutes.

Wild West Chili & Beans
Louisiana Red Beans & Rice
Thai Spicy Peanut Sauce w/Rice & Vegetables
Katmandu Curry w/Lentils & Potatoes
Shanghai Rice w/Vegetables
Sicilian Mixed Vegetables ❤
Green Beans Almondine
Diced Potatoes ❤
Peas ❤
Corn

The following dishes require minimal preparation:

Spaghetti and Sauce
Peas and Carrots ❤
Fruit Cocktail ❤
Oatmeal w/Mixed Fruit

Freeze-dried fruit selections contain only fruit:

Strawberries ❤
Peaches ❤

More Easy Travelin' Foods

PREFERRED BRANDS, INC.

Tasty Bite™ Indian Entrees
Just heat and eat these delectable dishes that come in handy, microwavable foil pouches. Bombay Potatoes ✍, Punjab Eggplant, and Madras Lentils.

Thai Table™ Thai Entrees
Authentic Thai meals come in foil pouches and are ready to serve in just minutes. Siam Green Curry with Vegetables, Bangkok Red Curry with Vegetables, Patong Yellow Curry with Vegetables, and Tom Yum Soup.

THE TAMARIND TREE, LTD.

Tamarind Tree — The Taste of India
The old world tradition of delectable Indian cuisine in microwavable/boilable trays accompanied by boil-in-bag brown rice. Now when I'm out of town with an Indian restaurant nowhere to be found, or it's 4:00 a.m. and I get a craving for spicy Indian cuisine, I thank the people at Tamarind Tree! Alu Chole ✍ (Curried Garbanzos & Potatoes), Channa Dal Masala (Golden Lentils with Vegetables), Dhingri Mutter (Garden Peas & Sautéed Mushrooms), Saag Chole (Tender Spinach & Garbanzos), and Vegetable Jalfrazi ✍ (Spicy Garden Vegetables).

For the Munchies

The best snacks are simple...fresh whole fruits, fresh-cut vegetables, nuts, seeds, trail mixes, or dried fruits and veggies. A few companies have made an art out of drying fruits and vegetables. They are included below. Also try air-popped popcorn sprinkled with Spike Salt-Free Seasonings or cinnamon.

BOULDER BAR ENDURANCE, INC.

Boulder Bar™
Tasty fruit juice sweetened, oven-baked real food energy bar snacks are high in complex carbohydrates and low in fat. Original Chocolate ❀ ✍, Boulder Berry ❀ ✍, Peanut Butter ❀, and Apple Cinnamon.

GOLDEN VALLEY FOODS

Advantage\10™ Whole Grain Fruit Bar
These chewy nutrition bars are made with real fruit and are low in fat and sodium. Cranberry Apple and Apple Cinnamon.

HEMPZELS

Hempzels Original Hemp Pretzels
These all natural pretzels are hand-rolled, hearth-baked, and low in fat. In Original, Black Pepper, Jalapeño, Garlic, and Onion.

THE JUST TOMATOES COMPANY

Just Tomatoes™ ❤
Like the name says, just tasty bits of vine-ripened, hand-picked tomatoes. As with all of the Just Tomatoes products, there are no salt, sulfur, sweeteners or preservatives added. In slices or crumbles, they are great sprinkled in salads!

Just Bell Peppers ❤
Just Carrots ❤
Just Corn ❤
Just Peas ❤

Just Veggies ❤ ✍
A wonderfully sweet and crunchy snack of carrots, corn, peas, bell peppers, and tomatoes. Eat it just like popcorn!

Hot Just Veggies ❤
The added jalapeño will make your tongue and taste buds sizzle.

Just Fruit Crunchies ❤ ❀ ✍
Apples, raisins, blueberries, sour cherries, mango, pineapple, and raspberries.

Just Fruit Snacks ❤
This fruit treat is chewy, not crunchy. Made with apples, persimmons, raisins, and pears.

Just Apples ❤
Just Persimmons ❤

Just Soy Nuts
Dry-roasted soybeans.

KALI'S SPORTNATURALS, INC.

Clif™ Bars
A natural energy bar made with rolled oats and packed with flavorful goodies. Chocolate Chip ✍, Crunchy Peanut Butter, Real Berry, Chocolate Espresso, Apple Cherry, Dark Chocolate, Apricot, Chocolate Chip Peanut Butter Crunch ❀ ✍, and Chocolate Almond Fudge ✍.

Kicks Bars ❀
The natural energy snack for both kids and adults! Peanut Butter Chocolate Chip, Strawberry, and Apple Cinnamon.

LENNY & LARRY'S

Lenny & Larry's Power Pops™ ❤
Tasty caramel coated air-popped corn that is fat-free and sweetened with Florida Crystals and rice syrup. In convenient snack-size packages and three fun flavors: Original ✍, Butter Toffee, and Chocolate Cappuccino.

MENTAL PROCESSES, INC.

Pumpkorn™ Alternative Snack Food ✍
Pumpkin seeds are a good source of omega-3 fatty acids and these flavor-charged treats will keep you wanting more. Original, Chili, Curry, and Maple Vanilla flavors.

NORTHERN LIGHTS HEMP CO.

Mama Indica's Hemp Seed Treats ⊕
Crunchy, chewy, nutty, sweet, and nutritious. Hemp seeds are a great source of protein and essential fatty acids. Four varieties: Hemp Seed Treats I with sesame seeds and nuts, Hemp Seed Treats II with sunflower seeds and nuts, Espresso Chocolate with whole espresso beans, and yummy Chocolate Raisin ✍.

Mama Indica's Roasted Hemp Seeds
Great for snacking or grind them and sprinkle over salads, soups, or stir-fries. Plain Roasted, Spicy (hot), and Eastern Hemp Seed Mix ✍ with lentils, rice crisps, cashews, peanuts, raisins, almonds, and spices.

ODWALLA, INC.

Odwalla Bar!
A tasty wheat-free energy bar made with fruits and grains. Cranberry Citrus and Peanut Crunch are vegan.

PAPAYA JOHN'S

Green Papaya Energy Bars ⊕ ✍
Sweetly delicious, these energy bars are a blend of green papaya with other fruits, nuts, bee pollen, and papaya honey concentrate. One small slice will give you an energy boost. Papaya & Fruit, Papaya Ginger, Papaya Almond, Papaya Sesame, Papaya Macadamia Nut, and Papaya Spirulina.

ROBERT'S AMERICAN GOURMET

Robert's Natural Snacks
Welcome to the future of snack food. Low-fat, healthy alternatives to traditional potato chips, corn chips, and

puffed doodles. Fruity Booty ✍ ❀, Veggie Booty ✍ ❀, Nude Food Caramel Corn, Nude Food Fra Diavlo Popcorn, Potato Flyers Original ❀, and Potato Flyers Pesto & Garlic.

Robert's Herbal Snacks
A uniquely delicious way to get your herbal fix. Cats Claw Crunch ✍, Ginkgo Biloba Rings, Kava Kava Corn Chips, Power Puffs w/Ginseng & Honey ❶ ✍, Spirulina Spirals, and St. John's Wort Tortilla Chips.

SUNDANCE COUNTRY FARM

Organic Dried Fruit ♥ ❀ ✍
The fruit, the whole fruit, and nothing but the fruit! The most succulently scrumptious, organic dried fruits, free of additives and sweeteners. Apple Rings, Apricots, Cherries, Figs, Peaches, Pears, Persimmons, Prunes (the best I've ever tasted), Raisins, Currants, and seven different varieties of Dates.

Organic Tropical Dried Fruit ♥ ❀ ✍
More sweet deliciousness. Whole Bananas, Pineapple, Mango, and Papaya (not certified).

TIMBER CREST FARMS

Sonoma® Dried Fruits ♥
With no preservatives or sulphur added, these dried fruits make wonderful snacks, can be sprinkled on cereal and salads, or be used in a wide variety of recipes. Persimmons, Cherries, Figs, Cranberries, Blueberries, Apples, Apricots, Peaches, Dates, Prunes, Pineapple, Star Fruit, Papaya & Mango, and Mixed Fruit.

Sonoma Dried Cosmic Squirrel Gorp™ ❀ ✍
A fabulously delicious super charged energy fix. This is an organic mix of almonds, apples, apricots, chocolate, coconut, dates, pears, prunes, and raisins.

Sonoma Dried Macho Mango™ ♥
Bits of mango showered in a mild chili and lime spice.

Sonoma Dried Tomato Bits ❤
Sprinkle on salads or blend into sauces and dressings.

Sonoma Crystallized Ginger ❤
Spicy-sweet golden nuggets are a refreshing nibble
any time of day.

— Chapter 5 —

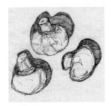

Burgers and Dogs and Meat Analogues

When you see the Golden Arches you're probably on the road to the Pearly Gates.
— William Castelli, M.D.

A few years ago, an obstinate friend of mine argued with me for hours on the pros and cons of eating meat (of course, there are no pros). I gradually convinced him that the high-cholesterol, high-fat content of his carnivorous diet was clogging his arteries and leading him on the fast track to a heart attack. He even admitted to me once that he knew that hamburgers didn't really grow in hamburger patches. But, he continued to eat meat because he insisted that he just couldn't deprive himself of the "pleasure." Like a wish come true, my friend came to me one day and promised that he would give up meat for a week if I could recommend acceptable substitutes. That is how this chapter was born. Happily, now all the "meats" he eats are from this list.

Meaty Tasting Burgers

AMY'S KITCHEN INC.

Amy's Organic Texas Veggie Burger ❶ ✍
The smoky barbecue flavor gives this burger a real "right off the grill" taste.

Key to Symbols: ♥ Fat Free ✍ Author's Favorite ❀ Kid's Pick
ⓒ Contains casein or caseinate ❶ Contains honey

BOCA BURGER COMPANY

Vegan Original Boca Burgers™ ❤ ❀ ✍
Textured like real hamburgers, and made from soy with a juicy, beefy, charcoal grilled flavor. Kids love 'em. A favorite at the White House and guaranteed to be a favorite at your house.

GARDENBURGER, INC.

Hamburger Style Gardenburger® ❤
New meaty flavored veggie patty from the makers of the original Gardenburger.

GOLDEN VALLEY FOODS

Advantage\10™ Mushroom Veggie Burger ✍
A pleasing combination of mushrooms, rice, onions, rolled oats, and seasonings give this burger a meaty flavor.

IMAGINE FOODS, INC.

Ken & Robert's Veggie Burger ⊖

LIGHTLIFE FOODS, INC.

Lightburgers™ ❀

VEGGIELAND

VeggieLand™ Veggie Griller
This soy-based burger boasts a truly meaty taste.

VITASOY, INC.

NewMenu™ Vegi~burger ❀
Terrific tasting.

WORTHINGTON FOODS, INC.

Morningstar Farms Better'n Burgers ❤
Original style only (others contain egg whites).

Natural Touch Vegan Burger™ ❤

YVES VEGGIE CUISINE INC.

Yves Veggie Cuisine® Burger Burgers ♥ ✿
Kids love 'em!

Great Veggie and Grain Burgers

AMY'S KITCHEN INC.

Amy's Organic California Veggie Burger
Wonderful hearty flavor from a nutritious blend of grains,
mushrooms, organic vegetables, and walnuts.

BLISS' SAN FRANCISCO

Bliss'™ Cafe Burger ✿ ✎
A scrumptious blend of grains, veggies, nuts, and soy give
this burger a distinctively satisfying taste.

FANTASTIC FOODS INC.

Nature's Burger
Four unique great-tasting flavors: Original Grilled,
Roasted Red Pepper and Garlic, Classic, and Southwestern
Black Bean ✎.

GARDENBURGER, INC.

GardenVegan™ ♥ ✎
Great veggie taste. It is similar to the original Gardenburger,
but without any animal ingredients.

GOLDEN VALLEY FOODS

Advantage\10™ Southwestern Vegetable Burger
A delightful medley of rice, beans, roasted bell pepper,
green beans, carrots, onion, corn, and soy seasoned with
zesty Southwestern spices.

MUD PIE FROZEN FOODS

Mudpie® Veggie Burgers
Straight from the menu of the famous Mud Pie Vegetarian
Restaurant in Minneapolis come these delightful burgers
made from such wholesome ingredients as brown rice,
tahini, fresh carrots, onions, oats, and millet.

SEENERGY FOODS LTD.

Nature's Chef™ Burgers
Loaded with spices and vegetables. Mexican Style Fajita, Mediterranean Style Falafel, and So Delight™ American Style Soy Bean ♥.

SUN FOODS LTD.

Sun's Veggie Light Patties
Delicious grain burgers. Choose from Rice ✍, Millet ✍, Bean, and Falafel varieties.

TURTLE ISLAND FOODS, INC.

Superburgers™
Juicy and full of flavor. Original, BarBQ ✍, and TexMex.

VEGGIELAND

VeggieLand™ Veggie Burgers
In two flavorful varieties: Original and Black Bean & Salsa.

WORTHINGTON FOODS, INC.

Natural Touch Hard Rock Cafe® Veggie Burgers ✍
The very same mouth-watering blend of sautéed vegetables, roasted nuts, mushrooms, and spices served in the famous worldwide restaurant chain. Also available under the Morningstar Farms label.

YVES VEGGIE CUISINE INC.

Yves Garden Vegetable Patties ♥

Yves Black Bean & Mushroom Burgers ♥

Tempeh Burgers

LIGHTLIFE FOODS, INC.

Lightlife Grilles®
Soy-rice tempeh burgers drenched in Barbeque, Tamari, or Lemon Marinade.

QUONG HOP & CO.

The Soy Deli™ All-Natural Tempeh Burgers
Delicious, precooked and ready in seconds. Original, Marinated, and Hickory BBQ ✍.

Tofu Burgers

Tofu burgers are traditionally high in fat. (Some get more than half of their calories from fat.) However, they are delicious and high in protein and other nutrients. When you do indulge, you may want to serve them on fat-free whole grain buns, along with a large, leafy green salad (with fat-free dressing), and oven-baked fries.

QUONG HOP & CO.

The Soy Deli All-Natural Tofu Burgers
Made with tasty tofu, vegetables, sesame seeds, sunflower seeds, and currants. Original, Garden, Teriyaki ❶ ✍, Texas BBQ ✍, Cajun Spice, Italian Spice, and Garlic Veggie.

WILDWOOD NATURAL FOODS

Tofu-Vegie™ Burgers
Made with tofu, onions, carrots, and kale. Also in Mexican, Italian, and Southwestern Wild West styles.

Unique Burgers

RELLA GOOD CHEESE CO.

Hempeh Burger
Unusual flavor made from nutrient-rich hemp seeds.

Hot Dogs

LIGHTLIFE FOODS, INC.

Smart Dogs® ❤
Taste just like hot dogs.

Smart Deli® Jumbos ❤
Smart Dog's big brother.

Tofu Pups®

Wonderdogs® ❀
A milder taste just for kids.

NORTHERN SOY, INC.

SoyBoy® Leaner Wieners™ ❤

SoyBoy Not Dogs
Made with organic tofu.

SoyBoy Right Dogs

QUONG HOP & CO.

Oh, my dog! ❀
For starters, you gotta love the name!

UNITED SPECIALTY FOODS

Longa Life™ notcorndogs™ ❀ ✍
A meatless frank in a yummy corn batter! A wonderful
treat for kids of all ages.

VITASOY, INC.

NewMenu™ VegiDogs ❤

WILDWOOD NATURAL FOODS

Wild Dogs ❤

YVES VEGGIE CUISINE INC.

Yves Veggie Wieners ❤ ❀

Yves Tofu Wieners ❤

Yves Jumbo Veggie Dog ❤
It's really, really big!

Yves Chili Dogs ❤ ✍
Nice spicy taste.

Chicken and Turkey Substitutes

GREEN OPTIONS, INC.

Vegetarian Slice of Life™ meatless "pull-apart" by Vegi-Deli™

Tasty chunks of flavored wheat protein you pull apart into desired portions. Use just like cooked meat: Marinate, sauté, grill, or toss into soups or salads. In Vegan Chick'n™ and Vegan Turk'y™ varieties.

HEALTH IS WEALTH, INC.

Chicken-Free Nuggets ❀ ✍

Made extra crispy, these tender nuggets are low in fat and breaded with stone-ground whole wheat. Superb new taste you can enjoy with your favorite dipping sauce: ketchup, barbecue sauce, honey mustard, or sweet and sour sauce.

Chicken-Free Patties™ ❀ ✍

Breaded with stone-ground whole wheat, these patties can be served on a bun, or add soy mozzarella and your favorite spaghetti sauce to make a delicious parmigiana dish.

NOW & ZEN, INC.

Breast of UnChicken™ ✍

Made with vital wheat gluten, yuba, herbs, and spices.

VEGGIELAND

VeggieLand™ Just-Like Chicken Marinated Cutlets ✍

Tender soy fillets are remarkably close to the real thing. Fully cooked and ready to use in your favorite recipe.

VeggieLand Just-Like Chicken Breaded Cutlets ✍

Ideal for making a delicious parmigiana.

VeggieLand™ Just-Like Chicken Breaded Nuggets ❀ ✍

Just heat and serve with your favorite dipping sauce.

VeggieLand™ Just-Like Chicken Strips ✍
Great for stir-fries, wraps, fajitas, and more.

Meat Analogues

These meat-alikes are great in chili, spaghetti sauces, and tacos.
They also make fabulous pizza toppings.

BOCA BURGER, INC.

Ground Boca Burger® Recipe Basics™ ❤
Seasoned, pre-browned, and packaged in easy-to-use
resealable bags.

EL BURRITO MEXICAN FOOD CO.

SoyTaco
A spicy meatless taco filling that really tastes great.

LIGHTLIFE FOODS, INC.

Gimme Lean!® ❤
Frozen ground meat substitute requires pre-browning.
Beef and Sausage ✍ flavors.

Meatless Smart Ground™ ❤
Ready to use beefy tasting crumbles for pizza, tacos,
stuffed peppers, and more.

Fakin Bacon Bits®
Great tastin' bits of fake bacon you can sprinkle over salads.
Made without any of the preservatives or artificial additives
commonly found in imitation bacon bits.

LUMEN FOODS

Heartline™ Meatless Meats
Great tasting assortment of styles have the look, taste, and
texture of a wide range of meats. Versatile and easy to use.
Requires no refrigeration. Just boil or microwave in water
for 15 minutes to reconstitute or snack on them right out of
the package! Plain Unflavored, Beef Fillet, Ground Beef,
Canadian Bacon, Chicken Fillet, Pepperoni, Italian Sausage,
Mexican Beef, Teriyaki Beef, and California Ham.

Heartline™ Lite
Lower in sodium and virtually no fat. Beef Fillet Style, Ground Beef Style, Canadian Bacon Style, Chicken Fillet Style, and Pepperoni Style.

NOW & ZEN, INC.

BBQ UnRibs™ ✍
Sensationally delicious!

THE SPICE OF LIFE CO.

Spice of Life Meatless Meats ✍
Easy, delicious, and versatile. Wide assortment of meatless meats require no refrigeration. Just add to boiling water for 10 to 12 minutes (6 to 8 minutes in microwave). Beef, Ground Beef, Mexican Beef, Teriyaki Beef, Chicken, Chicken Mince, Italian Sausage, Pepperoni, Smoked Ham, and Unflavored.

TREE OF LIFE, INC.

Ready Ground™ Tofu
Readily substitutes for hamburger in pasta sauces, chili, and much more! Prebrowned; just add to your favorite dish. In Original ✍, Savory Garlic, and Hot & Spicy.

WORTHINGTON FOODS, INC.

Morningstar Farms® Harvest Burgers for Recipes™ ❤ ✍
Pre-browned and ready to eat in clever zip-lock packaging.

Morningstar Farms Recipe Crumbles™
Textured vegetable protein and spices are precooked and recipe-ready. In Burger Style for use in tacos, sauces, and more.

Natural Touch® Vegan Burger Crumbles™ ❤

Natural Touch Vegan Sausage Crumbles™ ❤
Adds zest to lasagna, casseroles, and pizza.

YVES VEGGIE CUISINE, INC.

Yves Just Like Ground! ❤ ✍
Flavorful precooked premium meatless ground round.
Ready to eat, it comes refrigerated (not frozen) for added
convenience. In Original and Italian varieties.

Meatballs

VEGGIELAND

VeggieLand Veg•T•Balls™
Mama mia! These fully baked meatless meatballs boast a
real Italian taste. Look for them in your market's freezer
section.

Sandwich Slices

DELLA TERRA, INC.

Salami della Terra™ ✍
Sensational deli slices made with an old-world salami
technique using a unique combination of vegetables, fresh
herbs and spices, wheat protein, soy sauce, and water.
Whatever you have to do, get your hands on some of this
stuff! In six outstanding flavors: Texas Barbecue,
Southwestern Chili, Shiitake Mushroom, Yucatan Pepper,
Sundried Tomato, and Italian Pepperoni.

GREEN OPTIONS, INC.

Vegetarian Slice of Life™ meatless cold cuts from Vegi-Deli™ ✍
Delicious low fat, high-protein deli slices for making
hearty sandwiches that even true meat lovers will enjoy.
Made from wheat protein in Salami Style, Turkey Style,
and Chicken Style.

LIGHTLIFE FOODS, INC.

Foney Baloney®
Tastes like bologna, and that's no baloney!

Smart Deli® Slices ❤

Country Ham, Roast Turkey ✍, Old World Bologna, and Three Peppercorn styles.

TURTLE ISLAND FOODS, INC.

Tofurky™ Deli Slices ✍
Made with a revolutionary tofu-wheat protein combination that makes these slices taste fabulously delicious. In Original and Hickory Smoked flavors.

UNITED SPECIALTY FOODS

Longa Life™ Not Chicken™ and Longa Life™ Not Ham™
Tender sandwich slices imported from Australia.

WHITE WAVE, INC.

Meatless Sandwich Slices ❤ ✍
Chicken, Turkey, and Pastrami Styles.

YVES VEGGIE CUISINE INC.

Yves Deli Slices ❤ ❀
I never was big on luncheon meat, but I really do like these slices.

Yves Veggie Turkey Slices ❤

Sausage and Bacon

ALCALA ENTERPRISES

Maayo™ Natural Foods Vegetarian Chorizo™ ✍
Used in Mexican and Spanish cooking, chorizo is a highly seasoned, coarsely ground sausage flavored with garlic, chili powder, and other spices. This vegetarian version closely resembles the traditional sausage right down to the casing. Remember to remove the casing and crumble the chorizo before adding to tofu, pasta, or rice dishes.

Maayo™ Natural Foods Vegetarian Romanelli™ ✍
In Italy, romanelli refers to the best available meat in one's kitchen. By tradition, romanelli is saved for honored guests and special occasions. As in Italy, this vegetarian version is

seasoned with garlic, basil, and oregano. Remove the casing, sauté with onions, and crumble to add pizzazz to any of your favorite dishes.

EL BURRITO MEXICAN FOOD CO.

SoyRizo
This meatless soy chorizo made from textured vegetable protein is spicy and flavorful. Add it to tofu, stir-fried veggies, potatoes, chili, or rice dishes.

GREEN OPTIONS, INC.

Vegetarian Slice of Life™ Meatless Pepperoni from Vegi-Deli™
Sliceable little logs loaded with spices and boasting great texture. Tastes great alone, on a sandwich, or added to your favorite dishes. Ready to eat in Original, Zesty Italian, and Hot n' Spicy varieties.

LIGHTLIFE FOODS, INC.

Lean Links® Meatless Sausage
In Old World Italian Style and Country Breakfast Style.

Lightsausage®
All natural breakfast sausage patties.

Fakin' Bacon® Smokey Tempeh Strips ✐
Delicious organic soy tempeh strips. Heat and serve with scrambled tofu or use to make a BLT sandwich.

Smart Deli® Sticks ❤
Sliceable snack sticks that are great for picnics, snacking, or lunch on the run. Pepperoni and Three Pepper Soylami flavors.

NORTHERN SOY, INC.

SoyBoy Vegetarian Breakfast Links

THE PILLSBURY COMPANY

Green Giant® Breakfast Links

VEGGIELAND

VeggieLand™ Real Sausage Style Breakfast Links

YVES VEGGIE CUISINE INC.

Yves® Canadian Veggie Bacon ♥ ✍
Enjoy the traditional taste of Canadian bacon and rediscover the joy of an old-fashioned breakfast.

Yves Breakfast Veggie Links ♥
The first fat-free breakfast link!

Yves Veggie Pepperoni ♥

Yves Veggie Pizza Pepperoni ♥
Made especially to be used as a pizza topping.

Seitan

Seitan's versatility comes from its firm, chewy texture, which makes it an ideal substitute for meat (especially chicken). Also called wheat meat, seitan has a neutral taste. It easily picks up the flavors of the sauces, spices, and other foods with which it is cooked. The following seitan entries are ready to eat and can also be used in a variety of dishes.

LIGHTLIFE FOODS, INC.

Savory Seitan®
Premarinated and precooked wheat of meat dishes that are easy to heat and eat or slice and serve for great hot or cold sandwiches. With Barbeque Sauce ✍ or Teriyaki Sauce.

WHITE WAVE, INC.

Meat of Wheat Gourmet Grain Protein
Delicately seasoned, precooked tender chunks are great for salads, kabobs, sauces, and more. In Chicken Style only.

Traditional Seasoned Seitan ♥

Vegetarian Sloppy Joe

Snack Meats

GARDEN OF EATIN' INC.

Vegetable Jerky™ ❤
Smoky and chewy just like real jerky, in 3 flavors:
Hot n' Spicy BBQ, Pepperoni Pardner, and Western Roast.

LUMEN FOODS

Cajun Jerky
Beef, Hot Pepperoni, Spicy Italian, and Smoked Ham.

Stonewall's Jerquee
In Mild and Wild styles.

THE SPICE OF LIFE CO.

Spice of Life™ Meatless Jerky ✍
The ultimate vegetarian snack food. It's wonderfully
delicious.

Something's Fishy

WORTHINGTON FOODS, INC.

Tuno ❀ ✍
Tuno tastes, looks, and smells so much like tuna fish, the
first time someone offered it to me, I thought it was real tuna
and wouldn't eat it. Since then, my fears have subsided, and
I've become a real Tunoholic. Do with Tuno whatever you
would do with canned tuna. Mix it with a little Nayonaise,
celery, shredded carrots, onions, or relish. Spread it on whole
wheat toast and add a bit of leafy green lettuce and sliced
tomato. Then get set for an incredible lunchtime treat!
Although Tuno is now available in cans, it is very different
from the frozen variety. I highly recommend the Tuno found
in the freezer case.

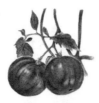

Chapter 6

Dressings, Dips, Sauces, and Spreads to Relish

Meat eaters are made, not born. The taste for fat and animal products can be readily changed.
— Charles Attwood, M.D.

You can enhance your health and well-being significantly by eliminating meat, dairy, and eggs from your diet. But, it is just as important to limit your intake of dietary fat. So, does that mean you have to give up rich tasting, dips, spreads, sauces and dressings? Absolutely not! Certainly, a fat is a fat is a fat, and as far as your waistline is concerned, one fat is as fattening as any other. Joyfully, many of the following condiments are completely fat-free or very low in fat and can be enjoyed frequently. Some items are high in fat, and should be used in moderation. However, all of the listings are free of unhealthful animal products, cholesterol, and hydrogenated oils. So, go ahead; pour, dip, schmear, and indulge yourself!

Key to Symbols: ♥ Fat Free   ✍ Author's Favorite   ❀ Kid's Pick
ⓒ Contains casein or caseinate   **ⓗ** Contains honey

Chutney

These traditional condiments from India add zestful flavor
to virtually any meal.

EARTH/SUN FARM

Earth/Sun Farm Chutneys
Made from organic ingredients grown in the small farming
community of Dixon, New Mexico. The delicate flavors of
these chutneys will delight your taste buds. Samadhi
Chutney ❶ ✍, Dixon Red Chile Chutney ❶, Southwest
Sunrise Apricot Chutney ❶, Urie Gingered Plum Chutney,
and Exquisito Piñon/Pear Chutney ✍.

ESSENCE OF INDIA, INC.

Essence of India™ Chutney ❤ ✍
Tomato Chutney is a provocatively sweet, spicy relish. Raisin
Chutney is tangy, fruity, and wonderfully delectable. Mango
Chutney is sumptuously savory and sweet.

GEETHA'S GOURMET PRODUCTS

Geetha's Gourmet Chutney ❶ ❤
Delicious Date & Raisin and Mango.

HAWAIIAN FRUIT SPECIALTIES LTD.

Hawaiian Kukui® Mango Chutney
With pineapples and assorted fruit flavors.

TAJ GOURMET FOODS

Taj Creative Condiments ✍
Tangy Tamarind Chutney, Sweet Mango Chutney ❶,
and Hot Mint Chutney.

WAX ORCHARDS INC.

Wax Orchards™ Chutney
Sweet and spicy condiments are sweetened only with fruit
juice concentrates. Apricot Ginger Chutney and Cranberry
Chutney ✍ (a great accompaniment to tofu turkey!)

Dips

I used to think a dip could mean only one thing: sour cream and onion soup mix. Then, all you needed were the potato chips. Talk about a fat and cholesterol laden snack! Now I know better. Dips can be fun, tasty, healthful additions to any party or you can enjoy them when you just feel like being a couch potato. The following dips are cholesterol and fat free. Just add fresh, cut fruits or veggies or your favorite baked tortilla chips and enjoy a totally guilt-free indulgence.

ASPARAGUS ENTERPRISES, INC.

Asparagus Guacamole ♥ ✍
A delightful fat-free version of a favorite Mexican snack food. Choice of Mild or Zesty.

GARDEN OF EATIN', INC.

Organic Fat Free Bean Dips ♥
Spicy Chipotle Red Bean ✍, and Baja Black Bean.

GOLDWATER'S FOODS OF ARIZONA

Goldwater's taste of the Southwest™ Black Bean Dips ♥
Fantastic concoctions of whole fruit and beans. Paradise Pineapple, Ruby Raspberry, and Mohave Mango.

GUILTLESS GOURMET, INC.

Guiltless Gourmet Fat Free Dips ♥
Mild Black Bean, Spicy Black Bean ✍, and Spicy Pinto Bean.

HUNGRY SULTAN MEDITERRANEAN GOURMET

Hungry Sultan™ Hummus
There's never been a more convenient way to enjoy hummus. These bean dips come in resealable little cans. Original, Spicy, Roasted Garlic, Cilantro, and Sun Dried Tomato ✍.

LITTLE BEAR ORGANIC FOODS

Bearitos® Fat Free Bean Dips ❤
Pinto Bean, Black Bean Salsa, and Black Bean.

MARANATHA NATURAL FOODS

Organic Sesame Tahini Hummus
These spicy Middle Eastern dips come in shelf-stable jars
and are great with pita bread, crackers, chips, or fresh
veggies. In three zesty flavors: Onion Cumin, Three Pepper,
and Lemon Garlic.

SAGUARO FOOD PRODUCTS

Saguaro No Fat Dips ❤
Spicy Black Bean ⓞ, Spicy Pinto Bean ⓞ, and Guacamole.
Also available under the Cool Coyote label at gift and
gourmet food shops.

SAHARA NATURAL FOODS, INC.

Casbah® Lemon Garlic Hummus
Garbanzo beans, tahini, garlic, and a touch of lemon give
this hummus packed in a jar a real Middle Eastern flavor.

Casbah® Baba Ganoush ✍
Now you can enjoy the taste of baba ganoush anytime.
It's made with eggplant, garlic, tahini, and lemon,
and comes in a shelf-stable glass jar.

SANTA CRUZ FINE FOODS

Santa Cruz™ Fat Free Guacamole ❤ ✍
Great taste made from spinach, corn, beans, and tomatoes
with just the right spices and seasonings.

Santa Cruz™ MediterrAsian Dip
A unique combination of hummus and wasabi.

Relish

When I discovered these relishes, I knew I had stumbled upon something exciting. You'll adore their unique, zesty flavors.

BIG SUR COAST FOODS

Naturally Smoked Red Pepper Relish ✍
The taste is sweet, not hot and can be used in sauces, dips, and spreads or try the fabulous recipe for "Mock Lox!"

QUICK TIP: MOCK LOX
Mix 1 cup of cream cheese alternative with 3 tablespoons of Naturally Smoked Red Pepper Relish. Spread on a sliced bagel. Add sliced tomato, onion, and a sprinkling of capers.

EARTH/SUN FARM

Earth/Sun Farm Eggplant Newcamp ❶ ✍
This wonderfully spicy, piquant relish will add pizzazz to any dish.

GEETHA'S GOURMET PRODUCTS

Fiesta Olé Hot Relish ❶ ❤
Try these relishes on salads, with crackers or chips, over your favorite veggie hot dog or mixed with Tuno. Hot Fruit and Hot Vegetable varieties.

Salad Dressings

BLANCHARD & BLANCHARD LTD.

Blanchard & Blanchard® Vermont
Classic Dressings
Mustard Vinaigrette, Lemon Pepper Vinaigrette, All Natural Poppy Seed, Honey Mustard Tarragon ❶, Toasted Sesame Seed, Northern Italian, Garlic, Tomato Basil, and Lemon Mustard Dill.

Blanchard & Blanchard® Vermont Fat Free Dressings ♥
Balsamic Tomato Herb, Balsamic Cracked Pepper,
and Balsamic Roasted Garlic.

Blanchard & Blanchard® Vermont Low Fat Spa Dressings
Balsamic Italian, Balsamic Honey Blackberry ❶,
Honey Dijon ❶, Country Italian, and Russian Tomato.

CARY RANDALL'S

Cary Randall's™ All Natural Sauces and Dressings
More than just dressings, these exciting condiments will
dress up pasta salads, steamed veggies, Tuno salad, and
more! Carrot Ginger Dressing ❶ ♥ ✍, Roasted Pepper
Vinaigrette ♥ ❶, Honey Mustard Dressing ❶ ♥, Roasted
Garlic Vinaigrette ❶ ♥, Hemp Pesto Vinaigrette ✍, Chile Out
Spicy Honey Mustard Dressing ❶ ♥ ✍, and Sundried Tomato
Basil Dressing ❶ ♥.

QUICK TIP: SPICY STEAMED VEGETABLES
Here's a flavorful dish without any fat:
Just add 1 teaspoon of water to a bowl of your favorite veggies, (try broccoli, carrots, or spinach). Top with 1 tablespoon of Cary Randall's Chile Out Spicy Honey Mustard Dressing and microwave for 3 minutes. Toss and enjoy!

DEL SOL FOOD CO., INC.

Briannas® Home Style Dressing
Available in supermarkets. Rich Poppy Seed ✍, Dijon Honey
Mustard ❶, Blush Wine Vinaigrette, Real French Vinaigrette,
and Zesty French.

Briannas Special Request Dressing ♥
Lively Lemon Tarragon ❶ and Rich Santa Fe Blend ✍.

FOOD FROM THE 'HOOD

Straight Out 'the Garden® Dressings
Delicious salad toppers from a natural food products
company owned and operated by inner-city high school
students. Creamy Italian and Honey Mustard ❶ ♥ ✍.

MARTIN BROTHERS CAFE

Martin Brothers Distinctive Salad Dressings ✍
Discover the vitality of the freshest of ingredients. Find
these dressings in your store's refrigerator case. Creamy
Miso, Tamari Vinaigrette, Garlic Mustard, and Thai Peanut.

MODERN PRODUCTS, INC.

Spike Splashers!™ Vinaigrette
From the makers of Spike Seasonings, three flavorful salad
dressing and marinade flavors. Splash them on salads,
stir fries, pasta, or rice dishes. In Original, Salt Free,
and Fat Free ♥.

NASOYA FOODS, INC.

Nasoya® Vegie-Dressing™
These creamy, full-bodied dressings will perk up your favorite
salad. Creamy Dill, Sesame Garlic, Garden Herb, Thousand
Island ✍, and Creamy Italian.

THE RAINFOREST COMPANY

Riverbank™ All Natural Dressings ❶
Fresh spices from the banks of the Amazon River create these
unique tasting dressings. 10% of The Rainforest Company's
earnings are donated to sustain the rainforest and its peoples.
Lime Vinaigrette ♥, Raspberry Cashew ✍, and Ginger Sesame.

SIMPLY DELICIOUS, INC.

Simply Delicious® Vinaigrette Un-Dressing
The secret to all the delicious flavor in these un-dressings
is Soy Gold™, a golden shoyu made with whole grains and
soybeans. Lemon Tahini, Miso Sesame ✍, Ginger Plum ❶,
Honey Mustard ❶, Tofu Poppyseed ✍, and Herb Garlic ❶.

herbalicious® Fat-Free Vinaigrette ♥
Made with organic apple cider vinegar: Garlic Italian,
Dill Cucumber, Miso Ginger, Tarragon Mustard **⊕**,
Tomato Basil **⊕**, and Roasted Pimento **⊕**.

SPECTRUM NATURALS, INC.

Spectrum Naturals® Dressing & Marinade
Zesty Italian, Mango Madness **⊕**, Sweet Onion & Garlic ♥,
and Toasted Sesame.

Salsa

Not just for chip-dipping, experience the amazing variety of salsas
available. They're great for adding spicy flavor to stir-fries, salads,
rice, pasta, or scrambled tofu dishes.

ADELINE'S GOURMET FOODS, INC.

Adeline's™ Gourmet Salsa ♥ ✍
Fruity and flavorful in three tantalizing varieties:
Mango, Kiwi, and Pineapple Guava.

ALLIED OLD ENGLISH, INC.

Sorrel Ridge® Fruit Salsa ♥
Boasts a fruity-tomato taste in mild or medium. Peach,
Orange Peel, and Pineapple ✍.

COYOTE COCINA

Coyote Cocina Salsa ♥
Created by world-famous chefs at the Coyote Cafe in Santa
Fe, New Mexico. Four unique flavors: Fire-Roasted ✍,
Roasted Corn & Black Bean ✍, New Mexico Green Chile,
and Flamin' Pineapple.

FLO'S DELICIOUS FOOD

Peach Walnut Salsa
A sweet and spicy combination of peaches, walnuts,
and chile. Dazzle your tastebuds with Mild ✍, Medium Hot,
and Very Hot varieties.

GARDEN OF EATIN', INC.

Organic Fat Free Salsa ❤
Cha Cha Corn ✍, Hot Habanero, and Great Garlic Mild.

GEETHA'S GOURMET PRODUCTS

Fiesta Olé Salsa ❤
Thick and hearty in Green Chile Bean and Red Chile Bean.

GOLDWATER'S FOODS OF ARIZONA

Goldwater's taste of the southwest™
From subtle and fruity to fiery hot! Sedona Red ❤,
Rio Verde Tomatillo ❤, Paradise Pineapple ❤, Ruby
Raspberry ❤, Sabino Strawberry ❤ ✍, Mohave Mango ❤,
Papago Peach ❤, Sedona Red Hot ❤, and Cochise Corn
and Black Bean ✍.

GUILTLESS GOURMET, INC.

Guiltless Gourmet Fat Free Salsa ❤
Medium Salsa, Green Tomatillo, Roasted Red Pepper,
and Southwestern Grill.

HAWAIIAN FRUIT SPECIALTIES LTD.

Kukui Tropics Hawaiian Papaya Salsa ❤
Unusual, distinctive taste with just a hint of curry.

Hawaiian Jungle Jazz Sweet & Sassy Guava Salsa ❤

KNUDSEN & SONS, INC.

R.W. Knudsen Family Fruit Salsa ❤
The sweetness of pineapple combined with peppers and
tomatoes for a truly unique taste. Available in two flavors:
Tomato & Pineapple and Pineapple & Pepper. In Mild ✍
and Hot varieties.

MILAGRO COUNTRY FOODS

Milagro™ Country Foods Salsa ❤
Spicy, hot, and delicious. Passion Peach and Habanero Fiesta.

NEWMAN'S OWN, INC.

Newman's Own All-Natural Bandito Salsa ♥
All profits go to charity. Comes in Mild ✍, Medium, and Hot.

THE RAINFOREST COMPANY

Riverbank Salsa
Mango ♥, Brazilian Red ♥, Black Bean & Corn,
and Tomatillo Chipotle.

RGE, INC.

Southwest Spirit™ Gourmet Culinary Salsa
Rio Red Habanero with Dried Tomatoes.

SAGUARO FOOD PRODUCTS

Saguaro No Fat Salsas ♥
Chipotle, Southwestern, and Santa Fe Harvest. Also available
under the Cool Coyote label at gift and gourmet food shops.

QUICK TIP: SASSY SALAD DRESSING
For a delicious fat-free or nearly fat-free salad dressing,
just pour your favorite salsa over tossed raw veggies!

SANTA CRUZ FINE FOODS

Santa Cruz™ Salsas ♥
Black Bean & Corn, Robust Red Amigo,
and Roasted Garlic & Red Pepper.

Sauces

BT TRADING COMPANY

Binz Jalapeño Ketchup ♥
Spice up your favorite veggie burger or dog with this jazzy
twist on traditional ketchup. In mild ✍, medium, and hot.

EDWARD & SONS TRADING CO., INC.

The Wizard's™ Vegetarian Worcestershire Sauce
A wonderful all-purpose, all-vegetarian condiment that will add zest to your favorite dishes.

ESSENCE OF INDIA, INC.

Essence of India™ Sauces
Bring home the savory flavors of India with Bombay Mint Sauce ♥ and Classic Curry Sauce.

GEETHA'S GOURMET PRODUCTS

Geetha's Gourmet Curry Sauces ✍
These thick, rich curries are packed with vegetables. Each variety is truly a meal in itself. Punjab Spinach or Vegetable Curry ♥.

HAWAIIAN FRUIT SPECIALTIES LTD.

Hawaiian Kukui® Sweet Sour Sauce
Zesty taste made with pineapples.

HOLY CHIPOTLE

Holy Chipotle ✍
A wonderfully spicy sauce made from chipotle peppers. Can be added to any Mexican food, used as a marinade, barbecue sauce, or just enjoyed with chips.

THE HOT TOMATO KITCHENS, INC.

Santa Fire™ Salsa Ketchup ♥ ✍
The perfect accompaniment to your favorite Southwestern bean burger.

HUNT-WESSON, INC.

Hunt's® Manwich® Sloppy Joe Sauce ♥ ❀ ✍
Fabulously fun food! Just add your favorite ground meat substitute from Chapter Five and serve on whole wheat buns. (I like using the Original flavor with Morningstar Farms

Harvest Burgers for Recipes™.) Original, Bold, Barbecue, and Taco & Burrito varieties.

THE RAINFOREST COMPANY

Riverbank™ Cooking Sauces
Exotic rainforest flavors add spice to tofu, tempeh, pasta, stir-fries and more! Mulitas Marinade ♥ (tangy, citrus Cuban Marinade), Jamaican Jerk (smoky and spicy), or Ginger Curry Stir Fry ❶ (with an Oriental accent).

RGE, INC.

Southwest Spirit™ Zia Fire
This fiery hot sauce combines the fresh flavors of habanero chile, garlic, peanut, and pineapple.

SIMPLY DELICIOUS, INC.

Flavors of the Rainforest™
Add exciting flavor to dishes with these new tropical condiments. Papaya Pepper Tropic Hot Sauce ❶, Green Habanero Hot Sauce ❶, Savory Spice Everyday, Everyway Sauce ❶, Ginger Curry Stir-Fry Sauce, Mango BBQ & Grille Sauce ❶, and Five Pepper Sauce ❶.

Troy's® Natural Saucery
Savory sauces create wholesome and natural international dishes. Low Fat Peanut Sauce ❶ (great for Thai dishes), Low Fat Garlic Sauce, Fat Free Curry Sauce ❶ ♥, Fat Free Jerk Sauce ❶ ♥ (for Caribbean flavor), Fat Free Chipotle Sauce ❶ ♥ (for Mexican and Southwestern meals), and Fat Free Ginger Sauce ❶ ♥ (for noodles and Oriental rice dishes).

TAJ GOURMET FOODS

Taj Simmer Sauces
Heat and serve sauces create the exotic flavors of India. Serve with vegetables and tofu over rice or with chapati or pita bread. Bombay Curry and Calcutta Masala.

Seasoning Sprays

GARLIC VALLEY FARMS

Garlic Juice Spray ♥ ✍
99.3% farm fresh, pure garlic juice to spray on salads,
pasta dishes, veggies, and soups. Also works great for
making garlic bread!

SPECTRUM NATURALS, INC.

Spectrum Naturals Seasoning Sprays ♥ ✍
A novel way to add seasoning to stir-fries, soups,
or grilled vegetables. Mediterranean or Asian flavors.

Spreads

ALLIED OLD ENGLISH, INC.

Sorrel Ridge® 100% Fruit ♥ ❀ ✍
Spreadable fruit sweetened only with fruit juice concentrates.
Blackberry, Strawberry, Black Cherry, Raspberry,
Boysenberry, Black Raspberry, Apricot, Wild Blueberry,
Peach, Concord Grape, and Orange Marmalade.

AMERICAN SPOON FOODS, INC.

Spoon Fruit® ♥ ❀ ✍
A delectably elegant gourmet collection of rich spreadable
fruit sweetened with fruit juices. Rich and luscious like
fruit spooned from a freshly baked pie. Sour Cherry,
Red Raspberry, Apricot, Peach, Blueberry, Strawberry,
Black Cherry, Apple, Blackberry, Cherry-Blueberry, and
Boysenberry.

Zingerman's® Blends Spoon Fruit® ♥
Cherry-Berry and Black and Blueberry.

American Spoon® Fruit Butter ♥
Fruit juice sweetened fruit butters will enhance bagels,
English muffins, toast, or waffles. Creamy, smooth, and
delicious. Apple, Marionberry, Cherry, and Red Raspberry.

American Spoon® Mango Butter ♥ ✍

Puréed mangoes sweetened with sugar and blended with pineapple juice, banana, and lime juice. A heavenly taste to die for!

American Spoon® Pumpkin Butter ♥ ✍

Sweetened with pure maple sugar and spiced like pumpkin pie, spread this sensational butter on a bagel, or serve warm over your favorite vanilla frozen dessert.

FOLLOW YOUR HEART

Vegenaise® Dressing & Sandwich Spread

The taste of real mayonnaise without the usual eggs, dairy, or refined sugars. Must be kept chilled to maintain its creamy, whipped texture, so look for it in your store's refrigerator case. Original, Expeller Pressed, and Grapeseed Oil varieties.

GALAXY FOODS CO.

Galaxy Foods® Veggie Margarine ☻

Lower in fat than traditional margarine and made with non-hydrogenated canola oil. Look for it in your supermarket's dairy case.

GREEN OPTIONS, INC.

GourMayo™

A wonderful vegan sandwich spread and dip in Classic, Dijon, Pesto ✍, Chipotle, and Garlic & Herb varieties.

THE HAIN FOOD GROUP, INC.

Hain Eggless Mayonnaise Dressing ☻ ✍

No added salt and high in vitamin E. Tastes very much like real mayonnaise.

HEALTH TRIP FOODS INC.

Health Trip Co. Soynut Butter ❀ ✍

A nut-free, soy protein-rich alternative to peanut butter with 33% less fat than natural peanut butter.

INTERNATIONAL BUSINESS TRADE, INC.

Marie Sharp's All Natural Jams ✍
Sensational exotic fruit spreads imported from Belize. Banana ♥ ❀, Coconut, Mango ♥, Papaya ♥, and Mixed Tropical Fruit ♥.

MCCUTCHEON APPLE PRODUCTS, INC.

McCutcheon's Home Recipe Fruit Spreads ♥ ❀ ✍
Fruit juice sweetened and packed with whole fruit. Black Raspberry, Whole Blueberry, Boysenberry, Whole Cherry, Cranberry Orange Marmalade, Grape Jelly, Orange Marmalade, Peach, Red Raspberry, Strawberry, Chunky Apple, and Blackberry.

McCutcheon's Home Recipe Fruit Butter ♥ ✍
Tongue tingly, smooth, with a delightful fruity taste. Sweetened with fruit juice. Apple, Pear, Cherry, and Pumpkin.

MRS. MALIBU FOODS, INC.

Peanut Better ❀ ✍
What's extraordinary about this peanut butter spread? It's 92% fat free! Now you can have it all. Great peanut butter taste and only 2.5 grams of fat per serving! Original, Berry Blast, and Chocolate Chunk flavors.

NASOYA FOODS, INC.

Nayonaise® Vegi-Dressing™ & Spread ✍
Creamy, delicious eggless alternative to traditional mayonnaise.

Fat-Free Nayonaise Vegi-Dressing & Spread ♥ ✍
Rich, full-bodied spread without the fat! How'd they do that?

THE PEACEWORKS, INC.

Moshe & Ali's Spratés™
Multipurpose sauce/spread/patés add zip to sandwiches, pasta, pizza, potatoes, or veggies. Sundried Tomato, Summer Garden, Basil Pesto, and Smoked Eggplant ✍ varieties.

POIRET INTERNATIONAL

Poiret no sugar added Fruit Spreads ♥ ✍

These specialty spreads imported from Belgium are made from pure fruit juices and nothing else. The juices of 7 pounds of fruit are packed into every 1 pound jar. In five fruity, sweet n' gooey flavors: Date & Apple, Pear & Apple, Pear & Apricot, Pear & Prune, and Pear, Apple, & Raspberry.

SOYCO FOODS

Rice™ Low Fat Spread ☯

Boasts a creamy, buttery flavor.

THE SOYNUT BUTTER CO.

I.M. Healthy™ SoyNut Butter ❀ ✍

A great tasting alternative to peanut butter made from fresh roasted soybeans. In three varieties: Creamy, Chunky, and 100% Organic.

SPECTRUM NATURALS, INC.

Spectrum Spread™ ✍

A marvelous tasting casein-free, non-hydrogenated, cholesterol-free alternative to butter and margarine. Original, Only Olive, Essential Omega, and Mediterranean varieties.

WAX ORCHARDS INC.

Wax Orchards Only Fruit™ Butter ♥ ❀ ✍

Scrumptiously smooth spreads boast an old fashioned flavor. Apple, Raspberry, Strawberry, Peach, Apricot, and Marionberry.

Wax Orchards Only Fruit™ Berry Spread ♥ ❀ ✍

Thick and fruity topping for toast or bagels or mix with soy yogurt! Made with whole berries. Blueberry, Marionberry, Strawberry, and Raspberry.

WORTHINGTON FOODS

Natural Touch® Roasted SoyButter™ ❀ ✍

Allergic to peanuts? Tired of nut butters that separate and turn hard? Roasted SoyButter has a rich, smooth, and creamy texture. A wonderfully nutty tasting alternative to peanut butter.

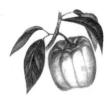

CHAPTER 7

Frozen Meals: Chilling Surprises

Eating vegetables and tofu will keep you in peace.
— Chinese folk saying

In my freezer I have an extraordinary assortment of international cuisine. I no longer feel that I have to eat at a restaurant in order to take my palate on a trip to faraway lands. From the classical, to the exotic, there is an abundant selection of taste-tempting frozen foods to explore.

American Favorites

AMY'S KITCHEN INC.

Amy's Vegetable Pot Pie ❶
Wholesome and hearty goodness.

Amy's Shepherd's Pie ✍
Organic vegetables simmered in broth and topped with mashed potatoes.

Amy's Macaroni & Soy Cheeze ❻ ❀
A real winner with kids!

Amy's Veggie Loaf Dinner ❶
Complete with mashed potatoes and a side of tender peas and corn.

Key to Symbols:	❤ Fat Free ✍ Author's Favorite ❀ Kid's Pick
	❻ Contains casein or caseinate ❶ Contains honey

THE HAIN FOOD GROUP, INC.

Farm Foods® Vegetarian Chili
Three varieties to choose from: Six Bean, Red Bean, and White Bean.

PHILCHIC, INC.

North American Recipe Vegetable and Brown Rice Pot Pie ☻
Baked in an organic whole wheat crust with crisp vegetables, beans, brown rice and Almond Cheeze™.

Indian Delights

Serve any of these flavorful dishes with the chutneys found in Chapter 6.

DEEP FOODS, INC.

Green Guru™ International Cuisine
Delicious Indian entrées: Channa Masala (chick peas sauteed with onions, tomatoes, and exotic spices), Vegetable Biryani ✍, (sautéed vegetables and tofu with savory sauce and exotic spices), and 4 Naan Bread, (traditional whole wheat bread is the perfect complement to Indian cuisine).

ETHNIC GOURMET FOODS

Taj Gourmet Meatless Authentic Recipes ✍
Delicately spiced classic Indian entrées served with organic rice pilau. Bean Masala (a delightful bean and tomato medley), Channa Bhajhi (sautéed chick peas with fresh ginger, garlic, and onions), Raj Mah (kidney beans sautéed with ginger, garlic, onions, and tomatoes), Eggplant Bhartha (roasted eggplant and green peas), Asparagus and Baby Carrots Subzi, Mushrooms and Green Peas Masala, Dal Bahaar (an aromatic blend of lentils and garlic with carrots, green peppers, and tofu), and Vegetable Korma (a mixture of fresh vegetables with ginger, garlic, tomatoes, onions, cashews, and raisins).

Taj Gourmet Samosas ❿
Savory Indian turnovers that are baked, not fried. Three zesty fillings to choose from: Aloo (potato), Gobi (cabbage and peas), and Subzi (mixed vegetables).

NATURAL LIFE, INC.

Jaipur Roti Express
Wheat tortillas filled with mildly spiced curried Indian vegetables. Try Bean Medley, Cauliflower and Peas, Mixed Veggies ✍, and Bombay Potatoes with Onions.

Jaipur Baked Vegan Samosa
Savory pastries stuffed with peas, potatoes, and mild spices.

Jaipur Entrees
Flavorful dishes served with Basmati Rice Pilaf. Vegan Chili, Madras Lentils ✍, Punjab Chick Peas, Lima Beans and Veggies, and Vegetable Melange ✍.

International Foods

CASCADIAN FARM

Cascadian Farm® Meals For A Small Planet™
Organic vegetarian meals with an international flair. Cajun, Oriental, Aztec, Moroccan ✍, Mediterranean, and Indian.

Cascadian Farm® Organic Veggie Bowls™
Szechuan Rice, Teriyaki Rice, or Pasta Marinara.

GLORIA'S KITCHEN

Gloria's Kitchen™ Jamaican Jerk Tofu

GOLDEN VALLEY FOODS

Advantage\10™ Entrees ✍
Recommended by Dr. Dean Ornish, these tasty dishes will please your palate and your waistline. Only 10% or less calories from fat and contain no artificial ingredients or

preservatives. Mediterranean Pasta, Caribbean Sweet'n Sour, Pasta Santa Fe, and Vegetable Szechwan.

LIGHTLIFE FOODS, INC.

Vegetarian Request® Meals
Five classic recipes: French Country Stew, Moroccan Lentil Stew, Tuscan White Bean Stew, Thai Tofu, and Traditional Meatloaf.

RUTHIES FOODS

Ruthies Complete Vegetarian Meals
Hearty and filling complete meal dishes in convenient boil-in-bags. Chili, Black Beans & Rice, Split Pea Soup, Adzuki Beans & Rice, and Lentils & Rice.

VEGGIELAND

VeggieLand™ Vegetarian Entrees 🖎
Uniquely delicious and satisfying dishes that will please even the most die-hard carnivore's palate. Southwestern Black Bean Chili, Stuffed Cabbage, Penne with Meatless Meat Sauce, and Meatless Loaf.

Italian Classics

AMY'S KITCHEN INC.

Amy's Tofu-Vegetable Lasagna ☺

CELENTANO

Celentano® Vegetarian Selects Non-Dairy Vegan Entrees
Delizioso! Eggplant Rollettes 🖎, Lasagna Primavera 🖎, Spinach & Broccoli Manicotti 🖎, Spinach & Broccoli Stuffed Shells 🖎, Eggplant Medallions with Garbanzo Bean Filling, Eggplant Wraps with Three Bean Filling 🖎, Roasted Vegetable Lasagna, Vegan Eggplant Parmigiana 🖎, Penne with Roasted Vegetables, Porcini Risotto with Roasted Vegetables, and Risotto with Eggplant, Tofu, and Spinach.

GLORIA'S KITCHEN

Gloria's Kitchen™ Tofu Balls & Spaghetti

THE HAIN FOOD GROUP, INC.

Hain Pure Foods® Vegetarian Classics
Radiatore Bolognese (cooked pasta in marinara sauce).

HEALTH IS WEALTH, INC.

Pizza Supreme Wraps ☻
Meatless pepperoni, sausage, and soy mozzarella cheese
wrapped in stone-ground whole wheat crust.

HKS MARKETING, LTD.

Legume® Fine Vegetarian Cuisine
Italian classics you'll savor: Stuffed Shells, Classic Lasagna,
Manicotti Florentine, Vegetable Lasagna, and Classic
Manicotti.

HOT MAMAS' RAVIOLI, ETC.

Hot Mamas' Large Spinach Tofu Ravioli ✍
Packed with tofu, spinach, carrots, onions, garlic, and spices.

NORTHERN SOY, INC.

SoyBoy® Ravioli ✿ ✍
Made with organic tofu. Too delicious for words.

SoyBoy Ravioli Verde™
Spinach pasta with garden-herb filling.

SoyBoy Ravioli Rosa™
Tomato pasta with roasted sweet pepper filling.

SEENERGY FOODS INC.

Casalinga Tofu Ravioli ✍
Filled with tofu and teeny-weeny pieces of mixed vegetables.

Knishes

GABILA AND SONS MANUFACTURING, INC.

Gabila's™ Potato Knishes ✍
"The original Coney Island Square Knish" is 99% fat free!
Also available in Spinach and Mixed Vegetable varieties.

HKS MARKETING, LTD.

Legume® Potato Pockets
A knish by any other name would still taste as great!
Potato, Spinach, and Broccoli.

R.F. BAKERY INTERNATIONAL, INC.

Klassic Knishes ✍
You'll plotz once you try any of one these baked potato
pockets in seven fabulous flavors: New York Style Potato,
Mediterranean Style Spice Potato, Mushroom & Garlic,
Broccoli, Spinach, Kasha, and Sundried Tomato.

Mexicana Olé!

AMY'S KITCHEN INC.

Amy's Burritos
Breakfast Burrito, Bean & Rice Burrito, and Black Bean
& Vegetable Burrito.

Amy's Black Bean & Vegetable Enchilada ❀ ✍
Organic corn tortillas filled with a medley of organic
vegetables, black beans, tofu, olives, and peppers topped
with a traditional Mexican sauce.

Amy's Black Bean & Vegetable Enchilada
with Spanish Rice & Beans ❀ ✍
A complete enchilada dinner.

Amy's Mexican Tamale Pie
Organic pinto beans, corn, zucchini, and crushed tomatoes
covered in a cornmeal polenta topping.

CEDARLANE NATURAL FOODS, INC.

Cedarlane™ Low Fat Beans, Rice, & Cheese Style Burrito ☻ ☻
Made with soy cheddar cheese.

Soypreme Tofu Enchilada Dinner ☻
With Spanish brown rice and refried beans.

GOURMET TAMALES

Gourmet Tamales™ ✍
Like no tamales you've ever tasted! Homemade goodness
shipped to you frozen and ready to eat in less than five
minutes in your microwave. Tomatillo Salsa, Chipotle Salsa,
Spicy Potato in Banana Leaf, Spicy Mushroom-Garlic, Green
Mole & Vegetables, Corn, Scallion, & Jalapeño, Red Mole-
Green Beans, Potato-Cilantro, Spinach-Zucchini, and
Roasted Red Bell Pepper-Chipotle Sauce.

NATURE'S HILIGHTS, INC.

Soy Cheese & Vegetarian Bean Tostada ☻
Completely gluten and yeast free.

TUMARO'S HOMESTYLE KITCHENS

Tumaro's™ Burritos
Three delicious varieties are microwave-ready in just three
minutes. Black Bean, Non-Dairy Cheese ☻, and Beans, Rice
& Potatoes.

Taste of the Orient

AMY'S KITCHEN, INC.

Amy's Asian Noodle Stir-Fry
Tender organic rice noodles combined with mushrooms,
water chestnuts, and vegetables in a traditional Chinese
brown sauce.

DEEP FOODS, INC.

Green Guru™ International Cuisine
Flavorful Thai delights. Vegetable Pad Thai (tangy and spicy stir-fried rice noodles with vegetables, tofu, spices, and ground peanuts) and Vegetable Gaeng Daeng ✍ (mixed vegetables and tofu with basil, lime leaves, red curry, and coconut milk).

DISCOVERY FOODS

Ling Ling® Vegetable Potstickers ✍
Plump little dumplings filled with cabbage, tofu, onions, water chestnuts, green beans, and carrots. Comes complete with dipping sauce.

Ling Ling® Veggie Curry Manapua ✪ ✍
Manapua are a traditional Hawaiian delicacy eaten for breakfast or enjoyed as an all-day snack. These delicious steamed vegetable buns are filled with a delightful medley of diced vegetables in a sweetly spiced curry sauce.

ETHNIC GOURMET FOODS

The Thai Chef™/Ethnic Gourmet Rice Bowl Meals
Pad Thai with Tofu ✍ is a traditional Thai specialty of rice noodles in peanut sauce with tofu, scallions, and carrots. Vegetarian Teriyaki has baby corn, water chestnuts, snow peas, carrots, and green peppers sautéed in an authentic Teriyaki sauce over long-grain white rice.

The Thai Chef™ Entrees
Sweet & Sour Vegetables are a medley of vegetables and pineapple sautéed in a tangy sweet and sour sauce. Thai Massaman Curry ✍ has bamboo shoots, tofu, mushrooms, red pepper, celery, carrots, and onions sautéed in an authentic vegetarian curry sauce. Both are served over jasmine rice.

GLORIA'S KITCHEN

Gloria's Kitchen™ Oriental Entrees
Orange Peel Soy Chick w/Organic Brown Rice, Mu Shu
Vegetables, Hoisin BBQ Vegetables w/Organic Noodles,
Spicy Thai Pumpkin Curry, Spicy Thai Tofu Spinach
w/Peanut Sauce, and Spicy Kung Pau Vegetables w/Organic
Brown Rice.

HEALTH IS WEALTH, INC.

Health is Wealth® Egg Rolls
Hand-rolled with stone-ground whole wheat flour. Broccoli
Tofu **☉**, Pizza Tofu **☉**, and Spinach Tofu **☉** have a delicious
soy-cheesy taste. Vegetarian ✍, Oriental Chicken-Free ✍,
and Oriental Vegetable ✍ styles are casein-free.

Health is Wealth® Steamed Dumplings ✍
Stuffed with a delectable assortment of vegetables, tofu,
and pineapple. This is a bit of dim sum heaven. Serve with
soy dipping sauce, "duck" sauce, or hot mustard.

LUCKY FOOD CO.

Lucky Pan-Fried Noodles

Lucky Spring Rolls ✍
These are delectable, authentic tasting little spring rolls.

SUN FOODS LTD.

Sun's Veggie Light Oriental Dumplings ✍
Scrumptious appetizers will remind you of dinner at your
favorite Chinese restaurant.

Pizza

AMBERWAVE FOODS

Soydance Pizza **☉** ✿
Crispy organic whole wheat crust with a tofu mozzarella
cheese topping.

AMY'S KITCHEN INC.

Amy's Roasted Vegetable Pizza ⑪
Tasty cheeseless pizza with organic shiitake mushrooms, artichokes, and roasted bell peppers.

ETHNIC GOURMET FOODS

Bravissimo!® Pizza ⑪ ✍
Grilled cheeseless pizzas overflowing with a bounty of vegetables. Roasted Vegetable and Spicy Thai Vegetable.

GOLDEN VALLEY FOODS

Advantage\10™ Roasted Vegetable Pizza ⑪ ✍
A crunchy whole-grain crust layered with roasted red and green bell peppers, onions, mushrooms, and olives topped with a thick and hearty spicy tomato sauce. Low in fat and high in flavor!

THE HAIN FOOD GROUP, INC.

Farm Foods Pizsoy Pizza ⊙
Made with an organic whole-wheat crust. Try Original, Fat-Free Cheese Style ❤, Fat-Free Garden Style ❤, and Fat-Free Vegetarian Pepperoni ❤.

NATURE'S HILIGHTS, INC.

Rice Crust Soy Cheese Pizza ⊙
Completely gluten- and yeast-free.

TREE OF LIFE, INC.

Special Delivery™ Organic Pizza ⊙
Made with Soya Kaas™ soy cheese.

Pockets and Wraps

Pockets and wraps are pastries stuffed with a variety of fillings. They are a great alternative to soup when you feel like a hot, quick, and satisfying lunch.

AMY'S KITCHEN INC.

Amy's Pocketfuls™ Vegetable Pot Pie ❶
Stuffed full of organic vegetables and tofu.

IMAGINE FOODS, INC.

Ken & Robert's Veggie Pockets
Ten delicious varieties baked in wholesome organic wheat crust: Greek ❸, Pizza ❸ ❀, Oriental, Tex-Mex ❸, Indian ✍, Potato and Cheddar ❸, Pot Pie, Santa Fe ❸, Broccoli and Cheddar ❸, and Bar-B-Que ✍.

CEDARLANE NATURAL FOODS, INC.

Cedarlane™ Low Fat Veggie Wraps ❶
Rice & Vegetable Teriyaki.

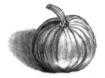

CHAPTER 8

Fun Foods for Parties, Holidays, and Special Occasions

...Earth is generous
With her provision, and her sustenance
Is very kind; she offers, for your table,
Food that requires no bloodshed and no slaughter.
— Ovid

The entries featured in this chapter are truly worth celebrating. Delight your family on holidays (or any day) with a healthful and delicious tofu turkey. Impress your party guests with elegant hors d'oeuvres, pâtés, and smoked tofu sensations. And when you want to savor the taste of down-home goodness while letting someone else do the cooking, try any of the homemade edibles recommended here. With the help of the foods in this chapter, you will be able to turn any meal into a delectably elegant, ambrosial affair.

Thanksgiving Feast

FRESH TOFU, INC.

Tofu Turkey™
A flavorful rosemary herb gravy mix accompanies these hand-scored, marinated, and freshly baked tofu "birds."

Key to Symbols:	❤ Fat Free ✍ Author's Favorite ❀ Kid's Pick
	● Contains casein or caseinate ❶ Contains honey

A fun way to celebrate Thanksgiving. Each Tofu Turkey serves 9.

NOW & ZEN, INC.

The Great UnTurkey™ ✍

Five pounds of delicately flavored seitan, dressed in a remarkable imitation turkey "skin" made from yuba and stuffed with a savory bread stuffing. Comes complete with a scrumptious gravy and serves 8. Seasonally available for the holidays at local natural food markets through the end of December.

TURTLE ISLAND FOODS, INC.

Tofurky™

A prebaked, vegetarian stuffed tofu roast turkey with dark tempeh drumettes and golden gravy. Available by special order through natural food stores or by calling Turtle Island direct. Serves 8.

QUICK TIP: A THANKSGIVING TO REMEMBER
Except for the bird, the Thanksgivings you've always enjoyed have been predominantly vegetarian affairs. Along with a stuffed tofu or seitan turkey, serve a large tossed salad, cranberry sauce, sweet potatoes, gravy, and green beans. Top it off with a tofu pumpkin pie and begin a tradition of truly memorable, delicious, healthful, and compassionate holiday celebrations.

Pâté

D'ARTAGNAN, INC.

D'Artagnan Vegetable Terrine ✍

Whether you are planning an elegant dinner party, want to entice your friends, or just treat yourself to something truly special, enjoy this scrumptious and gorgeous terrine. The three colorful layers of wild mushrooms, roasted red bell pepper, and spinach will please even the most refined palate. This rich pâté is available in upscale gourmet food specialty shops or you can order direct from D'Artagnan. Warning: this product is addictive *and* expensive, (but worth it!)

LIBERTY RICHTER INC.

Bonavita Vegetarian Pâté
Imported from Switzerland in Garlic and Herb varieties.

Smoked Tofu

Sliced thinly and placed on a cracker, smoked tofu is reminiscent of the taste of smoked gouda cheese.

TREE OF LIFE, INC.

Tree of Life® Smoked Tofu
Organically grown soybeans and a fabulous, true smoked flavor in Original and Hot 'N Spicy ✍.

WILDWOOD NATURAL FOODS

Organic Smoked Tofu ⊕
Long hours of marination and basking in Wildwood's smoke house, give this tofu a superbly creamy texture and rich mellow flavor. In Mild Szechuan ✍ or Garlic Teriyaki flavors.

Hors d'oeuvres

COWBOY CAVIAR

Cowboy Caviar® Vegetable Caviar ✍
A succulent blend of eggplant, tomatoes, onions, and bell peppers. Serve this "poor man's caviar" atop a cracker or baguette round, as a dip for crudité, or as a stuffing for mushroom caps. In Original Style and Jalapeño Style (great as a dip for tortilla chips.)

GLORIA'S KITCHEN

Gloria's Kitchen™ Won Ton
Tasty won tons stuffed with vegetables and tofu in a flavorful hot and sour sauce.

HEALTH IS WEALTH INC.

Health is Wealth® Munchees
These bite-size taste treats are like miniature egg rolls. PizzaTofu ©, Broccoli Tofu ©, Spinach Tofu © ✍, Mexican Tofu ©, Pepperoni Style ©, and Pizza Supreme Style © ✍ are made with soy cheese. Veggie ✍ style is casein-free.

Health is Wealth® Potato & Onion Pierogies ✍
Little whole-wheat pockets filled with potatoes and spices.

Health is Wealth® Potstickers ✍
Plump little dumplings in crispy whole-wheat wrappers pack a sensational Oriental flavor. Pork-Free, Chicken-Free and Vegetable varieties.

VEGGIELAND

VeggieLand™ Sweet n' Sour Veg•T•Balls™ ✍
Meatless meatballs topped with a tasty tart 'n tangy sauce.

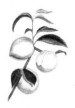

CHAPTER 9

Desserts: Ice Dreams and Beyond

Nothing will benefit human health and increase chances for survival on Earth as much as the evolution to a vegetarian diet.
— Albert Einstein

I love the expression, "Life is unpredictable; eat dessert first." Since I have been known to dream about pastry, I am forced to admit that this is often my mantra. Unfortunately, most traditional "goodies" are made with dairy products and eggs, so they are loaded with saturated fat and cholesterol. Here, I dedicate an entire chapter to all of my fellow dessert lovers. If you have been looking for animal-free alternatives with which to satisfy your sweet tooth, you've come to the right place.

Brownies

ALLISON'S COOKIES

Allison's Heavenly Fudge Brownies ❋ ✑
A bit of vegan heaven delivered right to your door.
Lusciously rich and chocolaty.

Key to Symbols: ♥ Fat Free   ✑ Author's Favorite   ❋ Kid's Pick
ⓒ Contains casein or caseinate   **ⓗ** Contains honey

FRANKLY NATURAL BAKERS

Vegan Decadence Brownies
They're as devilishly delicious as the name implies.
Mocha, Chocolate ❅ ✍, Raspberry ❅ ✍, Peanut Butter ❅,
and Carob.

Vegan Decadence Blondies
Chocolate, Butterscotch, and Caffé Latte
(made with organic coffee).

SEASON'S HARVEST

Nantucket Brownies
Temptingly tasty. Chocolate Fudge, Mocha Fudge,
and Peanut Butter Fudge varieties.

SUNDANCE SWEETS

Sundance Sweets™ Brownies
Scandalously rich, chewy, and delicious. Black Bear Mocha,
Hint O' Mint, and Raspberry Kodiak Bear ✍ (if this is death
by chocolate, I'm ready to go!)

Chocolate Candies

You won't find any wimpy milk chocolates here. Just rich, deep,
dark chocolate sensations. Chocaholics beware! The following listings are highly habit-forming.

CHOCOLATE DECADENCE

Chocolate Decadence ✍
Sinfully delicious gourmet chocolates for serious chocolate
lovers. Pure Dark Chocolate Wafers, Chocolate Covered
Mixed Fruit, Chocolate Covered Roasted Nuts, Chocolate
Covered Organic Pretzels, and Chocolate Espresso Buttons
(made with ground espresso beans).

Chocolate Decadence Dairy-Free Truffles ✍
Too delicious for words. In Espresso, Amaretto, Rum,
Raspberry, and Cherry flavors.

CHOCOLATE EMPORIUM

Chocolate Emporium Non-Dairy Confections ✍
An array of dark chocolate confections too numerous to list
here. Everything from raspberry-filled hearts (sensational!)
and chocolate dipped strawberries to hand-rolled truffles and
chocolate covered pretzels. Gifts for every occasion include
heart-shaped chocolate boxes and chocolate swans. A few
items contain egg white, so be sure to ask when ordering.

CLOUD NINE, INC.

Tropical Source® Organic Chocolate Bars
Dairy-free and delicious in ten innovative flavors: Sundried
Jungle Banana ✍, Java Roast, Hazelnut Espresso Crunch,
Green Tea Crisp, Wild Rice Crisp ❀, California Raisins
& Currants ❀ ✍, Mint Candy Crunch, Red Raspberry
Crush ❀ ✍, Maple Almond Granola, and Toasted Almond.

DOLPHIN NATURAL CHOCOLATES

Dolphin Natural Chocolates™
Hand-made and malt-sweetened individual chocolate delights
wrapped in pretty foil paper. A portion of profits benefit
environmental organizations. Mint Crisp ✍, Organic Peanut
Butter ❀, Solid Dark Chocolate, Roasted Almond, Espresso
Nut, and Cashew Coconut Raisin ✍. Also enjoy chocolate
dipped pineapple, apricot, and papaya!

GHIRARDELLI CHOCOLATE COMPANY

Ghirardelli Dark Chocolate Bar

Ghirardelli Dark Chocolate Bar with Raspberries ✍
As enticing as it sounds!

THE RAINFOREST COMPANY

Sweet River Chocolates™
Distinctively smooth texture in four delectable flavors:
Chocolate, Raspberry ✍, Rainforest Crunch®, and Dark
Chocolate & Espresso.

RAPUNZEL PURE ORGANICS

Rapunzel™ Organic Swiss® Chocolate Bars
Great tasting chocolates sweetened with Rapadura™
(unrefined, evaporated sugar cane juice) and boasting a
distinctly adult taste. Semisweet Swiss Chocolate, Semisweet
Swiss Chocolate with Almonds, Semisweet Swiss Chocolate
with Hazelnuts, Bittersweet 70% Cocoa Swiss Chocolate, and
the Rio™ bar (Bittersweet Swiss Chocolate with Almonds).

NEWMAN'S OWN ORGANICS

Newman's Own™ Organics Chocolate Bars
Sweet Dark Chocolate Bars in Plain, Espresso,
and Orange flavors.

SUNSPIRE

Sunspire® Natural Chocolate Earth Balls
Make every day Earth Day with these foil-wrapped
chocolate sweeties.

Sunspire® Natural Sweets-to-Go™
Gourmet dark chocolate confections in convenient resealable
tubs. Organic Chocolate Almonds, Organic Coconut
Haystacks ✍, Organic Jumpin' Java (with real espresso
beans), and Organic Peanut Clusters.

Chocolate Mousse

NOW & ZEN, INC.

Chocolate Mousse HipWhip™ ❅ ✍
Lusciously delicious all natural dessert with a heavenly

rich, chocolate flavor and a light, fluffy texture. Top with HipWhip™ dessert topping!

Cookies

ALLISON'S COOKIES

Allison's Cookies ✍
Taste these fabulously scrumptious cookies and you'll think you've died and gone to vegan heaven! Made with the freshest organic ingredients and unrefined sweeteners. You can even request your cookies baked wheat-free. Available exclusively through mail order by calling Allison's Cookies. Once you've tried them, you'll literally salivate every time you see your mailman. Mint Chocolate Chip ❀, Lavender Lemon, Cardamom Pecan, and Snickerdoodles ❀ (cinnamon and sugar). Also try Allison's delectable Lemon Oat Squares.

ALTERNATIVE BAKING COMPANY, INC.

Alternative Baking Company Vegan Cookies
Sensuously rich and chewy delights taste more like cake than cookies. These new flavors are totally free of wheat, dairy, eggs, and hydrogenated oils. Choco Cherry Chunk ❀ ✍ is decadently chocolaty. SnickerDoodle is cinnamony sweet. P-Nut Fudge Fusion is made with real peanut butter and cocoa. HulaNut ✍ is a tropical blend of macadamia nuts, coconut, mango, and pineapple.

AMERICAN NATURAL SNACKS

Mi-Del® GingerSnaps
Old fashioned "Swedish Style" cookies boast a snappy ginger taste!

BARBARA'S BAKERY, INC.

Barbara's® Bakery Homestyle Cookies ♥
Moist, chewy, and fruit juice sweetened. Chocolate Mint, Oatmeal Raisin, Chewy Chocolate, and Nutt'n Crispies.

Barbara's Bakery Fat Free Fig Bars ❤ ✍
Whole Wheat, Wheat Free, or Raspberry.

Snackimals™ Animal Cookies ✿
Chocolate Chip, Vanilla, and Oatmeal-Wheat Free.

FRANKLY NATURAL BAKERS

Frankly Natural Cookies & Squares
Dairy-free, wheat-free, and tasty energy snacks or dessert
treats. Made with tahini, sesame, and sunflower seeds.
Cookies: Rice, Coconut ✿ ✍, Apricot-Almond, Raisin ✿,
Tahini, Chocolate Tahini, and Rainforest. Squares: Currant,
Pecan, Cashew-Apricot, Carob, and Date-Nut.

THE HAIN FOOD GROUP, INC.

Chocolate Animal Grahams ❶ ✿

Peanut Butter Animal Grahams ❶ ✿

HEALTH VALLEY FOODS, INC.

Original Oat Bran Graham Crackers ❶

J&J SNACK FOODS CORP.

PretzelCookie™ ✿
It's a pretzel! It's a cookie! No, it's a tasty twist in cookies.
Lemon, Ginger, Vanilla, Oatmeal, or Chocolate.

JACQUI'S GOURMET COOKIES, ETC.

Jacqui's Gourmet Cookies ✿ ✍
Sensationally moist, chewy, and delicious! Chocolate Chip,
Fudge Brownie, Cinnamon Raisin, and Lemon Sesame.

LADY J INC.

Lady J Original Cookies
Tasty cookies sweetened with fruit juice and available in
several varieties. Originals: Peanut Butter Pecan ✿, Date

Pecan ✍, Oatmeal Raisin ❀, Chocolate Chunk ❀ ✍, Orange Pineapple, Puffed Brown Rice, Apple Cinnamon, and Banana ❀. Wheat Free: Chocolate Chocolate Chunk ✍ and Date Almond. Lites: Cinnamon Lites, Chocolate Lites, and Oatmeal Date Lites.

MRS. DENSON'S COOKIE COMPANY, INC.

Mrs. Denson's Reduced Fat Cookies
Wheat free and fruit juice sweetened in Chocolate Chip Macaroon ❀ ✍, Quinoa Macaroon ✍, Date Walnut, Oatmeal Raisin ❀, and Chocolate Chip ❀ ✍.

Mrs. Denson's Organic Cookies ❀ ✍
Chocolate Chip.

NANA'S COOKIE COMPANY

Nana's Cookies ✍
The original "feel good cookie" is a high-carbohydrate energy food that really tastes great. Oatmeal Chocolate Chip ❀, Oatmeal Raisin ❀, Oatmeal Sunflower, Mild & Wild Carrot Ginger, and Double Chocolate Supreme ❀. Oatmeal Chocolate Chip and Oatmeal Raisin also come in wheat-free varieties.

NATURAL OVENS OF MANITOWOC WISCONSIN

Natural Ovens Cookies
Tasty cookies with all natural ingredients that are good for you, too. Made with oats, sunflower seeds, wheat germ, and flax. Oatmeal Raisin and Chip Mate (carob chips and coconut).

NEW MORN, INC.

New Morning® Natural Grahams ❶
In four varieties, these graham crackers boast a buttery taste. Honey, Ginger, Cinnamon, and Chocolate.

OREAN'S EXPRESS, INC.

Sistah's® Cookies ❶
Chocolate Carob Chip and Oatmeal Raisin ✍.

SEASON'S HARVEST

Boston Cookies
These chewy, delicious oversized cookes come in 6 varieties and can be delivered to your door. Oatmeal Raisin ✍ ❀, Chocolate Chip ✍ ❀, Peanut Butter ❀, Chocolate Chocolate Chip (doubly rich), Mocha Chocolate Chip, and Coffee Chocolate Chip.

ST. AMOUR

Rocks N' Rolls
These truly unique "French munching cookies" are hard, crunchy, and not overly sweet. Great for dipping in tea, grain beverage, hot cocoa, or eating alone. Lemon Vanilla, Orange Chocolate Chip, Brandy & Chocolate, Cinnamon ✍, Chocolate Peanut Butter Chip, and Raspberry Chocolate ✍.

TREE OF LIFE, INC.

Small World™ Animal Grahams ❀ ✍
Graham cracker cookies made without hydrogenated oils are fashioned in the shapes of endangered species. For kids and adults alike. Plain and Chocolate Chip varieties.

Cookie Lovers™ Creme Supremes ❀ ✍
The first all natural chocolate sandwich cookie to taste like an Oreo™. Also in Mint and Royal Vanilla flavors.

Fat-Free Cookies ❶ ♥
Golden Oatmeal Raisin and Harvest Fruit & Nut.

Dessert Tamales

GOURMET TAMALES

Gourmet Dessert Tamales™ ✍
Homemade dessert tamales (yum!) shipped right to your door. Pineapple-Raisin, Strawberry-Apple, Orange-Mango, Pumpkin-Spice, and Peach-Ginger flavors.

Dessert Toppings

HAWAIIAN FRUIT SPECIALTIES LTD.

Hawaiian Kukui® Fruit Syrups ✍
These tropical fruit syrups are simply sensational. Pour them over your favorite frozen dessert. They also make delicious toppings for pancakes and waffles! Guava, Coconut, Passion Fruit, Pineapple, Mango, Papaya, and Macadamia Nut.

NEWMARKET FOODS, INC.

Fat-Free Chocolate Ecstasy™ ❤
A rich tasting, dark chocolate topping. Very smooth and delicious.

NOW & ZEN, INC.

HipWhip™ ❀ ✍
You won't believe this amazing whipped topping that's definitely cooler than cool! Fruit juice-sweetened, made without any hydrogenated oil and only 7 calories per serving. Absolutely delicious over frozen desserts, puddings, pies, cakes, waffles, fruit gelatin, hot cocoa, and more!

RGE, INC.

Southwest Spirit™ Seductive Dessert Salsas
Drizzle these toppings over frozen "ice dreams" or cakes and indulge yourself in dessert heaven. Made from sweet fruits, brandy, and a hint of chile. They turn ordinary desserts into a lusciously exotic taste experience. Brandied Cherries Diablo, Brandied Apricots Diablo, and Brandied Chocolate Raspberries Diablo ✍.

WAX ORCHARDS INC.

Wax Orchards™ Fudge Toppings ❤
Spoil your tastebuds with these scrumptious fudge toppings made from concentrated fruit juices and Dutch cocoa. Spoon over frozen dessert, fresh strawberries, bananas, or dried fruit. Classic Fudge ✍ is a bittersweet treat and Oh, Fudge! ❀

has a rich, dark chocolate profile. Also try: Fudge Fantasy, Peppermint Stick Fudge, and Amaretto Fudge ✍.

Wax Orchards™ Fruit Syrups ❤ ❀ ✍
Enjoy these pourable berries over frozen desserts, waffles, or pancakes! Strawberry, Blueberry, Raspberry, and Marionberry.

Frozen Desserts

Many of these desserts closely resemble the ice creams they imitate in both taste and texture. They are great in sundaes, floats, or drizzled with syrup. For an outrageously decadent change of pace, try topping any of these frozen treats with the dessert salsas listed on page 97. Best of all, you can joyfully serve these desserts to your delighted children because you will know that they are completely free of animal-based ingredients.

IMAGINE FOODS, INC.

Rice Dream® Non Dairy Dessert
Cappuccino, Carob, Carob Almond, Cherry Vanilla, Chocolate, Chocolate Chip, Cocoa Marble Fudge, Mint Carob Chip, Orange Vanilla Swirl ❀ ✍ (tastes just like a creamsicle!), Strawberry, Vanilla, and Vanilla Swiss Almond.

Rice Dream® Supreme
Great new flavor sensations: Cappuccino Almond Fudge, Cherry Chocolate Chunk ✍, Chocolate Almond Chunk, Chocolate Fudge Brownie ✍, Double Espresso Bean, Mint Chocolate Cookie ✍, Peanut Butter Cup ❀, and Pralines N' Dream.

Rice Dream® Pies ❀ ✍
Two oatmeal cookies with a malt sweetened carob or chocolate coating. Vanilla Dream Pie w/Carob, Mocha Dream Pie w/Carob, Chocolate Dream Pie w/Chocolate, and Mint Dream Pie w/Chocolate.

Rice Dream® Bars ✿
Rice Dream dipped in malt sweetened chocolate or carob. Vanilla w/Carob, Strawberry w/Carob, and Chocolate w/Chocolate.

Rice Dream® Nutty Bars ✿
Rice Dream dipped in malt-sweetened chocolate and covered with peanuts. Vanilla or Chocolate.

Rice Dream® Cones ❶ ✿
Crunchy, chocolate lined cones filled with vanilla or chocolate Rice Dream and topped with peanuts and rich chocolate.

TOFUTTI BRANDS, INC.

Tofutti® Lowfat Non Dairy Frozen Dessert
Creamy 98% fat-free dessert sold in pints: Vanilla Fudge, Chocolate Fudge, Coffee Marshmallow Swirl, Strawberry Banana, and Peach Mango.

Tofutti Frutti™ Chocolate Dipped Pops ✿
Vanilla cream with Tutti-Frutti sorbet.

Tofutti® Teddy Fudge Pops ✿
The great taste of a real fudge bar!

Tofutti® Chocolate Fudge Treats ❤
Fat-free and sugar-free with real fudge taste!

TURTLE MOUNTAIN, INC.

It's Soy Delicious™
Fruit-sweetened creamy dessert in pints: Espresso, Awesome Chocolate ✿, Vanilla Fudge, Almond Pecan ✍, Vanilla, Raspberry, Chocolate Peanut Butter ✿, Espresso Almond Fudge, Chocolate Almond, and Carob Peppermint.

Organic Soy Delicious™ ✍ ✿
Creamy Vanilla and Chocolate Velvet flavors have created quite a stir among vegans who have missed the taste of

ice cream. Organic Soy Delicious has successfully achieved the rich creaminess of "real" ice cream without the use of hydrogenated fats. New to the market are three more great flavors: Chocolate Peanut Butter, Mint Marble Fudge, and Neapolitan.

Sweet Nothings™ Frozen Dessert ♥
Creamy and fruity flavors in pints: Black Leopard, Chocolate ✿, Chocolate Mandarin ✍, Tiger Stripes, Vanilla, Espresso Fudge, Very Berry Blueberry, Raspberry Swirl, Mango Raspberry ✍, and Piña Colada.

Sweet Nothings Sundae Bars ✿
Chocolate covered dessert bars: Chocolate/Vanilla Crunch flavor.

Sweet Nothings Fat-Free Bars ♥
Fudge, Mocha Mania, Passion Island, and Mango Raspberry.

Fruit Gelatin

Surprisingly few people really know what gelatin is made of. I'll never forget the time I was invited to a friend's home for Christmas dinner. There, sitting on the table at each place setting, was a compact little blob of opaque green goo, shaking and shimmying atop a curled lettuce leaf. When I politely declined to eat it, the hostess was clearly insulted and exclaimed, "But I made this especially for you!" Not wishing to dampen the joy of the season any further, I elected not to tell the hostess that animal bones, cartilage, tendons, hooves, and other slaughterhouse byproducts were used in making the shiny, green globules. I simply didn't eat the one placed before me.

THE HAIN FOOD GROUP, INC.

Superfruits™ Dessert Mix ♥ ✿
A light and refreshing dessert gelatin that's bursting with fruity flavor and free of animal ingredients. Strawberry, Orange, Raspberry, and Cherry.

Pies

MOTHER NATURE'S GOODIES, INC.

Mother Nature's Goodies Fruit Juice Sweetened Pies
Succulent fruit-filled flavor in a whole-wheat flour crust.
Comes frozen and unbaked. Apple, Apricot ✍, Blueberry,
Boysenberry, and Cherry ✍.

NATURAL FEAST CORP.

Natural Feast™ Gourmet Streusel Pies ✍
Fabulous fruity fillings, and scrumptious pie crusts made
without hydrogenated oils. Packed frozen and unbaked, just
heat in your oven. No one will believe you didn't bake them
from scratch. Natural Apple, Cherry, Blueberry, Peach, and
Cranberry-Apple.

Pudding

DR. McDOUGALL'S RIGHT FOODS, INC.

Instant Rice Pudding
Tasty pudding in a cup with vanilla and cinnamon.
Just add boiling water!

GRAINAISSANCE INC.

Amazake Pudding
Naturally sweet and tasty. Almond and Chocolate ✍.

IMAGINE FOODS, INC.

Imagine Pudding Snacks ❀ ✍
Chocolate, Banana, Lemon, and Butterscotch.

MORINAGA NUTRITIONAL FOODS, INC.

Mori-Nu Mates Pudding & Pie Mix ❶ ❀ ✍
Simply blend with Mori-Nu lite tofu in your blender or food
processor for a sensationally rich and creamy dessert.
Note: These mixes contain a very small amount of coconut
oil. Lemon Creme and Chocolate.

WESTBRAE NATURAL FOODS

Westsoy® Pudding Cups
In Vanilla and Chocolate ❀ ✍ flavors.

QUICK TIP: DAIRY FREE TOFU WHIPPED CREAM
Combine 1 pound soft tofu, 1 teaspoon vanilla extract,
1 teaspoon almond extract, ¼ cup sweetener, and ⅛ cup
soy milk in a food processor or blender. Refrigerate before
serving, then dollop over brownies, pudding, or fruit-flavored
gelatin!

Scones

Season's Harvest
Enjoy these wonderful English-style pastries without the
butter and eggs traditionally found in scones. Cinnamon
Raisin, Chocolate Chip, Orange Currant, and Apple
Cinnamon.

Sorbet

I have not tasted ice cream in years and I no longer miss it. Why?
Because I fell in love with sorbet! It's delectably smooth, fruity, satisfying, and fat-free! (Chocolate-flavored sorbets contain a negligible amount of fat from the cocoa powder.) You can enjoy the
creamy, rich taste of sorbet without the guilt, bloat, and mucous-
forming side effects of frozen dairy desserts. Most sorbet is completely free of animal products, but make sure you check the label
for egg white. Some companies add it to their chocolate-flavored
sorbet. Of course, the sorbets featured here do not contain any egg
white.

ARTISAN FOODS

Paradisio Sorbet™
So packed with fruit (60%!) are these scrumptious sorbets that
they have all the creaminess and "mouthfeel" of ice cream. In

11 exotic flavors: Coconut ✍, Mango ♥ ✍, Chocolate ✍ ✿, Guanabana ♥, Mango Passion ♥ ✍, Mixed Berry ♥ ✿, Piña Colada ✍, Pineapple ♥ ✍, Raspberry ♥, Strawberry ♥ ✿, and Zarzamora ♥ ✍.

Paradisio Sorbet™ Bars ✍ ✿
Fresh fruity flavor on a stick. Strawberry ♥, Coconut, Mango ♥, and Chocolate.

Paradisio Sorbet™ Cups ✿
Single serving 3.5 ounce cups. Coconut, Guanabana ♥, Raspberry ♥, Mango Passion Fruit ♥, Piña Colada, and Strawberry ♥.

BEN & JERRY'S HOMEMADE, INC.

Ben & Jerry's Sorbet
Satisfying and delicious with bits of real fruit: Purple Passion Fruit ♥, Strawberry Kiwi ♥, Lemon Swirl ♥ ✍, Doonesberry ♥ ✿, Mango Lime ♥, and Devil's Food Chocolate ✿ ✍.

CASCADIAN FARM

Cascadian Farm® Organic Sorbet ♥
Raspberry, Strawberry, Blackberry, Peach, Chocolate, Mango, and Luscious Lemon™.

Cascadian Farm Organic Sorbet Bars ♥ ✿
Chocolate, Strawberry, Orange, and Raspberry.

DOUBLE RAINBOW GOURMET ICE CREAMS, INC.

Double Rainbow® Sorbet ♥
Silky smooth and creamy. Chocolate ✍ ✿, Marion Blackberry ✍, Raspberry ✿, Rainbow ✿, and Mango Tangerine.

DREYER'S GRAND ICE CREAM

Dreyer's Whole Fruit™ Sorbet ♥
Strawberry ✍, Raspberry, Lemon, Peach, and Mango Orange.

ESKIMO PIE CORPORATION

Real Fruit™ Chunky Sorbet ♥ ✍
Made with real fruit chunks! Red Raspberry, Lemon Peel, Georgia Peach, Mountain Strawberry, Tropical Blend, Wild Berries ❀, Ruby Red Grapefruit, Strawberry-Banana ❀, Cranberry-Raspberry, and Watermelon-Strawberry.

GLACIER GOURMET, INC.

Pascal's™ Premium French Sorbet ♥ ✍
All natural, silky smooth, sensuous taste. Strawberry, Lime, Passion Fruit, Raspberry, Lemon, Orange, Mango, Chocolate ❀, and Peach.

HOWLER PRODUCTS

Howler Rainforest Fruit Sorbet ♥ ✍
Delicious, creamy adventures for your mouth! Made from rare forest fruits, the purchase of which supports rainforest preservation projects. Guava-Strawberry, Passion Fruit, Mango, Primal Scream Coffee Bean! (a delicious way to stay awake), Caribbean Cherry, Guanabana, Dark Forest Chocolate, Tropical Tangerine, Mayan Blackberry, and Rainforest Raspberry with Acai.

INTEGRATED BRANDS INC.

Columbo Sorbet ♥
Wildberry ❀ ✍, Peach, Mango, Lemon, Strawberry, and Raspberry.

Columbo Sorbet Pops ♥ ❀ ✍
Wildberry.

TOFUTTI BRANDS, INC.

Tofutti® Sorbet ♥
Chocolate, Strawberry, Orange Peach Mango, Lemon, Coffee, and Raspberry Tea.

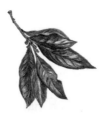

CHAPTER 10

Coffee Substitutes: Kicking Caffeine

What is this demilitarized zone? Whatever it is, I like it!
Gets you on your toes better than a strong cup of cappuccino!
— Robin Williams in *Good Morning Vietnam*

Have you been thinking about kicking the caffeine habit? Many people who eliminate meat from their diets find that they can no longer tolerate the "caffeine jitters."

There are also a number of health conditions for which doctors advise their patients to eliminate coffee. It is believed that caffeine may contribute to such problems as acid indigestion, anxiety, irritability and nervousness, fibrocystic breast disease, migraines or other vascular headaches, insomnia, and kidney or bladder problems. Caffeine also depletes the body of calcium. Therefore, if you are concerned about osteoporosis, it is advisable to limit your caffeine intake.

Following are delicious, naturally caffeine-free beverages that are rich enough to lure even the most confirmed coffee drinker.

Key to Symbols: ❤ Fat Free   ✍ Author's Favorite   ❀ Kid's Pick
© Contains casein or caseinate   **❶** Contains honey

Coffee Substitutes

ADAMBRA IMPORTS, INC.

Inka ♥ ✍

From Poland, an instant rich, natural-grain beverage made from roasted rye, barley, beets, and chicory root.

ALPURSA

Pero® ♥

Instant, natural-grain beverage from Germany made from barley, malted barley, chicory, and rye.

BIOFORCE OF AMERICA, LTD.

Bambu® ♥

A Swiss instant-grain beverage made with chicory, figs, wheat, malted barley, and roasted acorns.

CALIFORNIA NATURAL PRODUCTS

Dacopa™ Roasted Dahlia Powder ♥

A unique, full-bodied instant beverage made from the root of the dahlia flower. You'll notice a hint of sweetness from fructose that occurs naturally in the dahlia tuber. Dissolve in cold or hot water, or prepare with hot soy milk to make a tasty mocha-like drink that both kids and adults can enjoy.

I-D FOODS CORPORATION

Caf-Lib® ♥

An instant grain beverage produced in West Germany and imported from Canada. The Original Blend is made from roasted barley malt, barley and chicory. Dark Roast has rye and beet roots added.

INTERNATURAL FOODS, INC.

Cafix® ♥

Imported from Germany, this popular instant grain beverage is made from malt, chicory, barley, rye, figs, and beet roots.

KRAFT GENERAL FOODS, INC.

Postum® Instant Hot Beverage ❤
The original grain beverage introduced by C.W. Post over a century ago is still a popular favorite after all these years. Made from wheat bran, wheat molasses, and maltodextrin (from corn). In Regular and Natural Coffee Flavor.

LIMA

Yannoh ❤
A satisfying Swiss grain beverage made with organic barley, organic rye, organic malted barley, chicory, and acorns. Original and Vanilla flavors are available in instant and brewable varieties.

MODERN PRODUCTS, INC.

Instant! Sipp Natural Coffee Substitute ❤
Imported from Italy and made with 100% certified organic ingredients: roasted barley, chicory, rye, chick pea, and fig.

QUICK TIP: KISS CAFFEINE GOODBYE
When preparing your coffee drink, start with equal parts of coffee and instant grain beverage. Gradually reduce the amount of coffee and increase the amount of grain beverage each day. Soon you will find that you are enjoying a completely caffeine-free, flavorful alternative to coffee without the unpleasant side effects of caffeine withdrawal.

SUNDANCE ROASTING COMPANY, INC.

Sundance Barley Brew ❤
This savory beverage is brewed just like coffee—drip, perk, or espresso. Made from 100% organically grown barley.

TEECCINO CAFFÉ, INC.

Teeccino™ Caffeine-Free Herbal Coffee ♥ ✍

Now you can make scrumptious caffeine-free cappuccinos and lattés with this enticing herbal coffee made from carob, barley, chicory root, Persian figs, dates, and almonds. Teeccino is brewable, and boasts a rich, full-bodied flavor. Delicious hot or cold. The fragrant aroma is enticing. In Original, Almond Amaretto, Chocolate Mint, Vanilla Nut, Hazelnut, Java, and Mocha flavors.

WORTHINGTON FOODS, INC.

Natural Touch® Kaffree™ Roma ♥

Rich-tasting instant roasted-grain beverage made from roasted-barley malt, roasted barley, and roasted chicory.

Hot Chocolate

GHIRARDELLI CHOCOLATE COMPANY

Ghirardelli Hot Chocolates

Vegan hot cocoa mixes from heaven! Prepare with soy milk for a rich, creamy cocoa. Try Double Chocolate ❀ or Chocolate Hazelnut ✍.

Tea

There is an enormous array of wonderful tasting herbal teas available that are also naturally caffeine-free. However, most herbal teas will not satisfy a coffee drinker's craving for a rich, full-bodied beverage. Raja's Cup and Yogi teas are exceptionally rich and so amazingly satisfying that they live up to the challenge. The spicy taste of Oregon Chai makes it an exciting alternative to the daily grind. YerbaMaté is a unique herbal brew that will actually give you a boost of energy, too.

MAHARISHI AYUR-VED PRODUCTS INTERNATIONAL, INC.

Raja's Cup™ ♥ ✍

Brews like coffee, tastes like coffee, but it's good for you. Loaded with antioxidents that are reportedly hundreds of times more powerful than vitamin C or E. Made from rare and delicious Ayurvedic herbs for a rich-roasted flavor and it's 100% naturally caffeine free.

OREGON CHAI

Oregon Chai® Tea Latte ⓗ ♥

These sweet, spicy tea concentrates are a tasty alternative to coffee. Rich in flavor, the Original and Green Tea varieties have only 2 to5 mg. of caffeine per serving, compared to 35 to 50 mg. in a regular cup of tea or 128 to144 mg. of caffeine in coffee. The herbal blend is naturally caffeine-free. Mix with soy or rice milk for a sumptuously exotic hot or chilled beverage. Original Chai Latte is made with black tea, vanilla, ginger, and spices. Kashmir Green Tea has almond and ginseng added. Herbal Bliss ✍ is a soothing blend of chamomile, mint, and fresh spices. All are sweetened with honey.

QUICK TIP: HAZELNUT CHAI
Mix 60% Oregon Chai Tea Concentrate together with 40% Grainaissance Hazelnut Amazake. Heat and serve for a terrific tasting steamy beverage.

WISDOM OF THE ANCIENTS

YerbaMaté ♥

This amazing beverage has been a staple of the Guarani Indians of Paraguay for hundreds of years. Although tasting nothing like coffee, maté is the leaf of a South American evergreen holly. It contains the chemical mateine, which is similar to caffeine, but reportedly without many of caffeine's nasty side effects. It is said that you can give up coffee immediately by substituting maté tea. Claimed by many to be "the most powerful rejuvenator known to man" drinkers of maté enjoy increased energy without the intestinal problems or interruption of sleep cycles associated with coffee. Other reported benefits include acceleration of the healing process, relief from allergy symptoms, and fortification of the immune system. The non-addicting nature of maté makes it an excellent choice for those who want to kick caffeine.

Yerbamaté Royale™ ♥ ✍
A delicious blend of Yerbamaté, Licorice Pepper, and Honeyleaf™ Stevia that is naturally sweet. Yerbamaté Royale is reported to reduce the desire to smoke, especially when enjoyed through a "Bombilla" (metal straw).

THE YOGI TEA COMPANY

Yogi Tea™ ♥
These savory and exotic blends are available in tea bags to enjoy as quick, satisfying beverages, or by the pound for cappuccino, latté, or brewed iced spice tea. Tahitian Vanilla ✍, Carob Mint, Egyptian Licorice, Cinnamon Spice, Hazelnut Cream ✍, Mango Passion, and Maple Royale ✍.

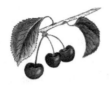

CHAPTER 11

Sugar Savvy:
The Scoop on Sweeteners

*How doth the little busy bee
Improve each shining hour,
And gather honey all the day
From every opening flower!*
— Isaac Watts *Divine Songs*

Did you know that it takes one bee her entire lifetime to produce just a single tablespoon of honey? This is one of the reasons vegans refrain from eating products that contain honey.

From a health perspective, honey, which is mostly made of glucose and fructose, is up to twice as sweet as white sugar. It enters the bloodstream rapidly, wreaking havoc on your blood sugar levels. Complex carbohydrates on the other hand, like those found in beans, fruits, vegetables, and grains are digested more slowly giving your body a more balanced sugar supply. Rice syrup and barley syrup are made of 50 percent complex carbohydrates and are therefore, better sweetening choices than honey.

It is important to note that honey may contain the toxin clostridium botulinum that can cause potentially fatal botulism. The levels present are not high enough to affect adults, but they can seriously affect infants. Therefore, children under the age of two should never consume any products containing honey.

Key to Symbols: ♥ Fat Free ✍ Author's Favorite ❀ Kid's Pick
ⓒ Contains casein or caseinate ⓗ Contains honey

Refined white sugar has almost no nutritive value, and contributes to many health problems such as obesity, tooth decay, and yeast infections to name a few. The fact that cattle bone char is often used in the refining process of white sugar makes it an ethical issue for vegans. The char is used to adhere to and help remove impurities from the raw sugar. However, manufacturers claim that it is somehow filtered out so that no ash remains in the finished product.

It is perfectly natural for humans to crave sweets. There is a significant amount of natural sugar in mother's milk, so we are born with this desire. However, artificial sweeteners are not suitable substitutes to satisfy your sweet tooth. Saccharin even comes with a warning label that it has caused cancer in laboratory rats.

By contrast, aspartame (Equal®, Nutrasweet®), comes with only one warning regarding the rare condition phenylketonuria that affects about 15,000 Americans. Since aspartame's introduction in the early 1980s, there have been thousands of consumer health complaints against it. There are ninety-two different complaints including gastrointestinal problems, headaches, rashes, depression, seizures, memory loss, blindness, slurred speech, and other neurological disorders. This should come as no surprise to the manufacturer of aspartame or the FDA whose own advisory committee recommended that it *not* be approved when laboratory tests indicated that aspartame produced brain tumors.

Aspartame is made of phenylalanine, aspartic acid, and methanol (wood alcohol). When methanol is ingested, it is broken down into formaldehyde. Aspartic acid is a neurotransmitter (a chemical used by the brain) and many experts believe that it causes brain lesions by literally exciting some brain cells to death, especially in children and older adults. Since aspartame's approval and introduction into over 4,000 food products, there has been a dramatic and sustained increase in the incidence of brain tumors with greater malignancy in the United States.

My own personal experience with aspartame is a story of ignorance turned to enlightenment. For years, I suffered from chronic, splitting migraine headaches at least four or five times a week.

I mainly attributed these frequent and painful episodes to a whiplash injury I had sustained in a car accident in 1986 (coincidentally, about the same time aspartame started flooding the market). When I finally started learning about aspartame's dangers and read that headaches were a frequent complaint, I threw out every piece of sugar-free chewing gum, container of Crystal Lite®, and little blue packet of sweetener in my kitchen cupboard. It has been more than a year now, and I have not had one single headache since I stopped consuming aspartame. Not one!

Yet another artificial sweetener, acesulfame k (marketed as Sunett® and Sweet One®) bears no warning label on its products. But laboratory studies showing lung tumors, mammary gland tumors, and premature death should be enough to stop anyone dead in his/her tracks from using it.

So, what's left? There is a broad spectrum of natural sweeteners to choose from with distinct health advantages over honey or refined white sugar. There's even an herbal sweetener that is hundreds of time sweeter than sugar, non-caloric, and safe for diabetics and hypoglycemics. As with all foods, always choose organic sweeteners whenever possible.

AGAVE NECTAR

A naturally sweet nectar from the blue agave plant, it's high in fructose and about 50 percent sweeter than refined sugar. The natural light variety is the ideal substitute for honey in tea. Its sweeter taste makes it a much more desirable choice than brown rice syrup or barley malt syrup. The darker variety is similar to molasses in taste and appearance, and is rich in natural minerals.

AMAZAKE

An oriental grain sweetener made from cultured brown rice. It has a thick consistency and is wonderful poured over cereals. When using amazake in baking, it adds a subtle sweetness, moisture, and leavening to recipes.

BARLEY MALT SYRUP

Made much like brown rice syrup, barley malt syrup uses sprouted barley to turn grain starches into a complex sweetener. It is dark brown, thick, and sticky, with a distinctive taste. It's half as sweet as refined sugar so it's best used in combination with other sweeteners in recipes. Adds a light sweetness to baked foods and is also available in granulated form.

BLACKSTRAP MOLASSES

This rich, dark syrup that is really nothing more than the "leftovers" from the sugar-refining process, marginally qualifies as a natural sweetener. Its most redeeming quality is that it retains most of the nutrients in the original sugar cane plant such as thiamine, niacin, riboflavin, calcium, iron, potassium, and magnesium. Blackstrap molasses has a very strong flavor and is a good choice when making quick breads, cookies, cakes, and pies.

BROWN RICE SYRUP

This is an amber-colored syrup made from brown rice starch that is converted into maltose. High in complex carbohydrates, brown rice syrup has the mildest flavor of all the liquid sweeteners. It can be used in baked goods or as a sweetener in hot beverages.

CRYSTALLINE FRUCTOSE

Derived from fruit sugar, this sweetener closely resembles granular white sugar, but is more concentrated, so less is needed. Almost twice as sweet as white sugar, yet provides balanced energy because it releases glucose into the bloodstream much more slowly. Not suitable in recipes requiring high temperature cooking, as heat causes crystalline fructose to break down.

DATE SUGAR

Made from dried, ground dates retaining many naturally occurring vitamins and minerals as well as fiber. Delicious when used in baked goods, or sprinkled as a topping over cereals and desserts.

DEVANSWEET™

A granulated organic brown-rice sweetener rich in carbohydrates. Ideal for use in cooking, baking, and hot or cold beverages.

EVAPORATED CANE JUICE/UNREFINED CANE JUICE

This is whole sugar cane with water removed. Minerals and molasses are retained and the cane is milled into granules of a light tawny color. The taste is milder than refined sugar with less sucrose (simple sugar). Suitable for use as an all-purpose sweetener.

FRUITSOURCE®

This sweetener is 80 percent as sweet as sugar, combining the sweetness of grape juice concentrate with brown rice syrup. Fruitsource replaces not only the sugar, but 50 percent of the fat, in baking. Available in liquid or granular varieties.

FRUIT SWEET®

A rich all-purpose liquid substitute for honey and sugar. It is sweeter than sugar, with 30 percent fewer calories. Made from pear, peach, and unsweetened pineapple concentrates. I prefer its sweeter taste to rice and barley syrup in tea. Wonderful in baking, as it adds moisture to any recipe. Fruit Sweet has been a sweetener of choice by the American Diabetic Association for many years.

GRAPE SWEET™

Concentrated grape juice is naturally sweeter than sugar or

honey. A lighter sweetener than Fruit Sweet®, it is ideal for making fruit preserves, cakes, and cookies.

MAPLE SYRUP

Containing small amounts of trace minerals, maple syrup has a rich taste and is absorbed fairly quickly into the bloodstream. Be sure to buy a pure, organic variety that does not contain added corn syrup.

STEVIA

Stevia rebaudiana Bertoni is a perennial shrub native to the Amambay Mountain region of Paraguay. It has been enjoyed by the Guarani Indians for hundreds of years, who use it primarily to sweeten their herbal maté tea. By the 1800s, daily consumption of stevia had spread to South American settlers in Paraguay, Argentina, and Brazil. In 1899, Stevia was "rediscovered" by Italian botanist, Moises Santiago Bertoni. This set the stage for the cultivation of stevia, which until that time had only grown in the wild of Paraguay.

The benefits of stevia as a sweetener are unrivaled:

• Stevia actually balances blood sugar levels, and is safe for use by both diabetics and hypoglycemics.

• Unlike aspartame, there are no reports of adverse effects from stevia's use and scientific studies throughout the world prove out its safety. Stevia has never been shown to cause brain tumors, seizures, blindness, or any of the other 92 adverse reactions reported to the FDA by users of aspartame.

• Unlike aspartame, stevia reduces the craving for sweets, making it the ideal sweetener for a society desperate to lose weight.

• Unlike sugar, stevia reduces cavities by retarding the growth of plaque.

- Stevia is used as a digestive aid in Brazil.

- Stevia contains antiseptic properties that have proven beneficial in speeding the healing process of skin wounds.

- Tests show that stevia's antimicrobial properties inhibit the growth of streptococcus and other bacteria. This is especially noteworthy since some forms of streptococcus have become antibiotic resistant.

Using stevia as a sweetener takes some adjusting. Stevia is so very powerful, (it can be 200 to 400 times sweeter than sugar) that you have to learn to use the smallest amount to achieve a desired sweetness. However, stevia's many benefits make learning how to use it an extremely worthwhile endeavor.

Currently, the FDA does not allow stevia to be sold as a sweetener in the United States. But don't wait for the FDA to give stevia its blessing. It may be a long time in coming. You can find stevia products in the supplements section of your local natural food store or refer to the index of this book for companies that ship stevia right to your door. I urge you to immediately (if not sooner) empty your kitchen cupboards of all products containing aspartame. Throw out your Equal®, Crystal Lite®, diet sodas, and chewing gum. Discard all toothpaste and children's vitamins that have aspartame listed on the label. You not only will become liberated, but a whole lot healthier in the process. And if you're ever again tempted to replace calories with chemicals, remember these words spoken eloquently by Julian Whitaker, M.D., "Frankly, I don't let aspartame into my house—children live there."

BODY ECOLOGY

Sweet 'N Better™ ♥ ✍
Stevia herbal concentrate in a convenient, pocket-size bottle that you can carry with you anywhere. Over 500 servings per bottle.

Stevia Powder Natural Herbal Extract ❤
The starter kit comes with 2 oz. of stevia powder, a dropper bottle, and an information booklet with recipes.

DEVANSOY FARMS, INC.

Devansweet™ ❤
Granulated organic brown-rice sweetener.

EDEN FOODS, INC.

Eden® Organic Malt Syrups ❤
Choose from Barley Malt, Rye Malt, and Wheat Malt varieties.

FLORIDA CRYSTALS, INC.

Florida Crystals ❤
Organic evaporated cane juice in two varieties. Milled Cane is a fine, golden color sugar with a delicate flavor. Demerara is a coarse grain sugar with a slightly sticky texture and a distinct molasses flavor. Great with hot beverages and cereals.

FRUITSOURCE ASSOCIATES

Fruitsource® ❤
An all-purpose sweetener and fat replacer made from grape juice concentrate and rice syrup.

GLORYBEE FOODS, INC.

Aunt Patty's Dry Sweeteners ❤
Granulated sweeteners in a wide selection of choices. Try Organic Maple Sugar, Organic Cane Sugar, Fructose, Date Sugar ✍, and Barley Malt Extract.

Aunt Patty's Brown Rice Syrup ❤

Aunt Patty's Barley Malt Syrup ❤

GRAINAISSANCE, INC.

Grainaissance Amazake
Available in original and a variety of flavors. See full listing on page 18.

NOW FOODS

Stevia Extract Packets ❤ ✍
Stevia extract powder in a rice maltodextrin base are packaged in handy sugar-like packets.

Stevia Extract Powder ❤

Stevia Liquid Extract ❤

NUNATURALS

NuNaturals Pure Liquid Stevia Extract ❤
Pure stevia extract in a base of vegetable glycerine and alcohol.

NuNaturals Pure Stevia Extract ❤
Highly concentrated.

NuNaturals Stevia Extract Powder ❤
Stevia extract in a maltodextrin base.

ONLY NATURAL, INC.

Fast Acting Stevia™ ❤
Pure stevia extract in a water base.

Steviaside™ ❤
Stevia extract leaves in a base of vegetable glycerin and water.

RAPUNZEL PURE ORGANICS

Rapadura™ Sugar ❤
Organic unbleached, unrefined evaporated sugar cane juice grown in Brazil.

STEVITA CO., INC.

Stevita® Spoonable Stevia ❤ ✍
A blend of 96% pure stevita crystals (stevioside) and corn maltodextrin.

Stevita® Packets ❤ ✍
Same as Spoonable Stevia in convenient, easy-to-carry packets.

Stevita® Powdered Crystal ❤ ✍
96% pure stevia powdered crystals without any filler. Very potent.

Stevita® Liquid Stevia ❤ ✍
Stevita powdered crystals in a base of distilled water. Comes in a handy bottle to carry in pocket or purse.

WHOLESOME FOODS

Organic Sucanat® ❤
Organic evaporated cane juice crystals blended together with organic blackstrap molasses. A tasty replacement for refined white or brown sugar.

Organic Plantation-Milled Sugar ❤
Unrefined cane sugar granules that retain a natural blond color and a delicately sweet taste.

Organic Blackstrap Molasses ❤
High in nutrients, robust in flavor, and not bitter tasting like some other varieties.

Organic Barbados Molasses ❤
Made from the first press of the sugar cane with a naturally sweet taste. It is lighter in color and flavor than blackstrap molasses and can be used to replace maple syrup in recipes.

WAX ORCHARDS

Fruit Sweet® ❤ ✍

Sensationally sweet tasting and versatile. Adds a wonderful moistness to baked goods and a delightful sweetness to hot or iced tea.

Grape Sweet™ ❤

Lighter than Fruit Sweet and just as versatile.

WESTERN COMMERCE CORP.

Cucamonga Organic Agave Nectar ❤ ✍

Grown organically in Mexico. Natural Light syrup is wonderful in hot beverages, and it's the perfect substitute for honey. Use Natural Dark syrup in recipes calling for molasses. Also available in powdered form.

WISDOM OF THE ANCIENTS

Stevia Extract Powder ❤ ✍

Great tasting, intensely sweet.

Stevia Extract Liquid ❤ ✍

Contains stevia extract powder in a water base.

Stevia Concentrate ❤ ✍

Highly concentrated, thick, rich, dark-brown liquid made by carefully cooking stevia leaves. Dilute for use in foods or beverages.

HoneyLeaf™ Ground Stevia Leaf ❤ ✍

Finely ground stevia leaves enhance the flavor of foods. A delightful licorice taste. Sprinkle over salads, soups, hot cereals, stews, and teas.

Stevia*Plus*™ ❤ ✍

A combination of sweet glycosides from stevia leaves and fructooligosaccharides (FOS), a prebiotic nutritional supplement. FOS is a mildly sweet low-calorie powder extracted from natural foods such as bananas, tomatoes, onions, garlic, and grains. Packaged in a 4 oz. bottle and in convenient individual packets.

Stevia Tea Bags ♥ ✍
Ground premium quality stevia leaves make a satisfying, naturally sweet hot or cold beverage.

WYSONG CORP.

Vegan Sweet Sensations ♥ ✍
A delicious, unrefined granulated sweetener balanced naturally to provide a broad spectrum of vitamins, minerals, and fiber. Combines cane sugar, stevia, and active food enzymes. Original Sweet Tooth™ can be used anywhere you need sweetening power: beverages, desserts, cereals, and baked goods. Cinnamon Ecstasy™ adds a touch of cinnamony sweetness to toast, cereals, or bagel spreads. Let your imagination go wild with Banana Delight™. Try Chocolate Craving™ in everything from soymilk to lattés. Lemon Quench™ is a naturally sweet lemon drink mix high in vitamin C.

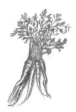

CHAPTER 12

The Pet Department:
Fluffy and Fido
Go Veggie!

*I care not for a man's religion whose dog
and cat are not the better for it.*
— Abraham Lincoln

The ugly truth about commercial pet food is that in addition to the high levels of toxic pesticides, chemical additives, and hormones that make up your pet's meat-based diet, you can add slaughterhouse waste, euthanized companion animals, and road kill to the menu. Many of the diseases that threaten the health of our pets may be directly related to their diets.

Dogs can easily adapt to an all-vegetarian diet. Cats, on the other hand, are true carnivores and require special nutrients typically found in a meat-based diet. Taurine, an essential amino acid, is manufactured in the bodies of all mammals except cats. They lack the ability to produce taurine and so they must get it from their diet, or succumb to blindness, disease, and death.

Fortunately, modern technology has helped researchers develop a process for extracting taurine from non-animal sources. The all-vegetarian cat foods listed in this chapter are supplemented with taurine and essential fatty acids that felines require for optimum health and well-being.

---

*Key to
Symbols:* ✍ Author's Favorite ❶ Contains honey

Like their human friends, companion animals benefit greatly from a diet that includes whole, fresh, organic foods. On such a diet, companion dogs and cats suffer far less from the rampant life-threatening diseases that afflict millions of pets whose food comes only out of bags or cans. You can easily incorporate whole, fresh foods into your pet's diet. I have included two easy vegetarian recipes in this chapter as examples of how to begin cooking for your animal companion.

Many argue that it is unnatural to "force" a cat or a dog to adopt a vegetarian diet. But, it is also not natural for these animals to consume the diseased carcasses of cows and sheep or other animals of their own species who have been euthanized and handed over to a rendering plant. Yet that is what our pets are most often subjected to when fed most commercial pet food.

Whether feeding your animal companion fresh foods or any of the commercially prepared vegetarian foods listed in this chapter, it is advisable to wean your pets off of their old diet by mixing a small amount of the new food with the old, and gradually adjusting the proportions over a period of days.

Both of my companion animals are life-long vegetarians. In fact, they are vegans, consuming no dairy or eggs. My cat, Indiana Jones, and my dog, Cicely Alaska, have enjoyed the best of health, beauty, and vigor. Your pets can thrive on a completely vegetarian diet too. If you cannot cook for your animal companions, at least try to supplement their diets with some fresh organic foods in conjunction with some of the following plant-based pet food products.

Canned Dog Food

EVOLUTION PET FOODS

Evolution™ Diet Dog Food
Formulated with wholesome and natural ingredients.
Peas & Avocado, Vegetable Stew, and Gourmet Pasta Flavor.

NATURAL LIFE PET PRODUCTS, INC.

Vegetarian Dog Formula

NATURE'S RECIPE PET FOODS

Vegetarian Canine Formula

PETGUARD, INC.

PetGuard® Premium Vegetarian Feast Dinner

Kibble for Dogs

EVOLUTION PET FOODS

Evolution Diet Pasta Seafood

NATURAL LIFE PET PRODUCTS, INC.

Vegetarian Dog Formula

NATURE'S RECIPE PET FOODS

Vegetarian Canine Formula

Dog Biscuits and Treats

AMERICAN HEALTH KENNELS

Bark Bars®
Fun, healthy treats shaped like mail carriers and cats.
Garlic, Peanut Butter, Carob & Peanut Butter, and
Wheat & Corn Free.

Jumbo Bark Bars®
A super-sized treat for your dog in the same great flavors
as original Bark Bars.

BOSS BARS

Willie & Tess' Boss of the House Bars
Made from 100% organic ingredients in Original and
Wheat & Corn Free varieties.

BRUNZI'S BEST, INC.

Brunzi's Best Doggie Divines
Unique organic treats. Can be wrapped for 9 different special occasions including Christmas, Chanukah, and Halloween. Biscuits come in Peanut Butter and Carob, Apple-Apricot, and Carrot-Cinnamon.

Potato Leek Canine Condiments ❶
These crumbled tasty bits can be sprinkled over food when Fido is feeling finicky.

DANDY DOGGIE

Dandy Doggie Gourr-met Dog Treats ✍
Gourr-geous gourr-met gifts for your favorite canine companion. This collection is made exclusively from organic whole wheat flour and other all natural ingredients. The treats are beautifully packaged and adorned with raffia, purple, and gold ribbons.

Biscotti per Bowser - A dozen assorted dog biscuits.

Bowownies™ - Carob flavored brownie squares.

Bowownies™ with Nuts

Bowser Brittle™ - Rainforest nut treat.

Bone-Anza™ - A very big bone.

New Chow Mein - Noodle-shaped treats come in a take-out carton complete with doggie chopsticks.

PowerBark™ - A nutritional snack bar just for dogs.

The Pound™ - A portion of the profits from these treats are donated to animal shelters, sanctuaries, and low-cost spay/neuter programs.

NATURE'S ANIMALS, INC.

Nature's Animals® All Natural Dog Biscuits
Handmade treats preserved with vitamin E. Peanut Butter and Vegetarian varieties.

OREAN'S EXPRESS, INC.

Mrs. Poochee's® Gourmet Cookies for Dogs
These big cookies look so tasty you'll be tempted to eat them yourself. Stop that! They're for your pooch.

PETGUARD, INC.

Mr. Barky's™ Vegetarian Dog Biscuits

PURR-FECT GROWLINGS

Purr-Fect Growlings® Dog Biscuit Treats
Simple ingredients in great tasting treats that are baked in the shape of the state of California and also in hearts.

ROBUSTO KITCHENS ✍

Robusto Biscotti di Cane™
These organic biscotti come in three flavors and three sizes. There's no wheat, corn, soy, preservatives, artificial flavors or colorings, so they're hypoallergenic, too. In Original Multi-Vegetable, Carob SweetPotato, and Vita Herb varieties.

WOW BOW DISTRIBUTORS LTD.

Pet Pastries, Gourmet Cookies
Gourmet line of freshly baked treats like bagels, snowballs, mini-croissants, and even birthday cakes. All vegetarian, many completely vegan. Call to receive their free catalog.

Canned Cat Food

EVOLUTION PET FOODS

Evolution™ Diet Cat Food
Healthy ingredients provide quality nutrients for your cat. Peas & Avocado, Vegetable Stew, and Gourmet Pasta Flavor.

Kibble for Cats

EVOLUTION PET FOODS

Evolution Diet Pasta Seafood
Completely vegetarian with added taurine.

Canine/Feline Kibble

WYSONG CORPORATION

Vegan™ Canine/Feline Diet ✍
Contains taurine and essential fatty acids cats require.
You can supplement your cat's diet with Vegecat™ to insure
the proper protein recommendations.

Dietary Supplements

Canine

HARBINGERS OF A NEW AGE

Vegedog™ ✍
Dogs are nutritional omnivores so they do not have the same
metabolic limitations as cats. But like humans, achieving the
proper nutrient balance in your dog's diet isn't always easy.
Vegedog takes away a lot of the guesswork. When used with
the recipes provided, which include whole, fresh foods from
your kitchen, you can be assured of meeting the dietary
recommendations for dogs.

Feline

HARBINGERS OF A NEW AGE

Vegecat™ ✍
Because cats are true carnivores, they need certain nutrients
like taurine that formerly only flesh foods could provide. If
cats don't get enough of this secondary amino acid (which
other mammals convert from the essential amino acids
methionine and cystine), they may become blind or suffer
from serious heart disease. Just add Vegecat to one of the

simple-to-prepare, veterinarian-approved recipes provided, and your cat can safely enjoy a completely cruelty-free diet.

Vegekit™ 🖎
A dietary supplement similar to Vegecat™, but specially formulated for kittens up to one year of age.

Dog Chews

ASPEN PET PRODUCTS, INC.

Booda Velvets™
Made from a revolutionary new-corn starch formula. Completely free of animal byproducts, preservatives, and toxins. In several sizes and flavors: Premium Mix, Chicken, and Beef & Vegetable.

NATURE'S RECIPE PET FOODS

EarResistibles™
A great low fat, non-meat alternative to pig-ear chews.

NYLABONE PRODUCTS

POPpup™ with Spinach
This potato starch-based Nylabone® chew is made with 100% edible, natural ingredients.

Nylabone® Corn-Bone
This edible chew is made with corn starch and potato starch. No animal ingredients. Both the POPpup and Corn-Bone come in a variety of sizes.

Vegetarian Recipes

GARBANZO SURPRISE*

(4 days food for a 10 lb. adult cat)
1 can garbanzo beans or 2 cups cooked beans
⅞ cup firm tofu
⅓ cup nutritional yeast powder
⅛ cup olive oil or high oleic safflower oil

½ teaspoon salt or 2 teaspoons soy sauce
4 teaspoons Vegecat™
Optional seasonings: garlic powder, tomato paste, etc.

Mix all ingredients together. Sprinkle with yeast before serving. Keep unused food in a covered container in the refrigerator.

LENTIL CHOW*

(2 days food for a 44 lb. adult dog)
3⅝ cups uncooked lentils
2½ tablespoons nutritional yeast powder
¼ cup safflower or corn oil
1 tablespoon Vegedog™
2 teaspoons salt or 2¼ tablespoons soy sauce
Season with garlic powder

Soak lentils in cold water for 2 hours. Drain, cover with water and cook until just soft. Thoroughly drain and add other ingredients. Sprinkle with yeast prior to serving. Keep unused food in a covered container in the refrigerator.

*Pet recipes are from *Vegetarian Cats and Dogs* by James Peden, (Harbingers of a New Age).

Cat Litter

Although cat litter is not an edible product, it may end up being eaten by your pet. So, I would like to share a discovery I recently made about conventional kitty litter. Like many people who enjoy sharing their homes with feline companions, I had become quite accustomed to the convenience of scoopable (clumping) litter. However, I did not know that clumping litter can be a deadly convenience for the cat. I learned how hazardous clay clumping litter can be only after my own cat got sick. And the dangers of clumping litter can even extend beyond your cat. If you have a dog who gets into the litterbox for occasional "snacks," then he or she will ingest the litter, too.

There are two main problems with clumping litter. First,

bentonite: the primary ingredient in clumping litters. Bentonite is a clay formed by the decomposition of volcanic ash that has the ability to absorb large quantities of water and to expand to several times its normal volume. After cats and kittens use the litterbox, they lick themselves clean and anything their tongues encounter gets ingested. Once some clumping litter gets inside a cat it expands and can form a mass (exactly what it is designed to do inside a litterbox—not inside your cat!). This causes dehydration and also prevents any absorption of nutrients or fluids.

Second, clumping litters and conventional clay litters both contain silica dust, a known cancer-causing agent. When poured into your cat's litter box, and kicked up by your cat, silica dust rises into the air posing the risk of bronchial and respiratory infections. Of course, humans and companion animals are both susceptible to inhaling the dangerous dust. Prolonged exposure to silica dust causes silicosis in humans and animals, a sometimes fatal lung disease. Fortunately, there are many wonderful safe, convenient, and effective alternatives.

AMERICAN NUTRITION

Natural Harmony® Premium Cat Litter ✍
This unscented "Pet•Pourri" is an all natural blend of wheat grass fibers in pellet form. Its super absorbency makes it superior at controlling cat box odors. It lasts twice as long as clay litters, is safe, dust-free, and flushable.

BLOSSOM PRODUCTS CO.

CitraFresh®
This product is 100% citrus and nothing more. Highly absorbent, biodegradable, and it has a naturally fresh scent. Lightweight and available through mail-order.

EARTHSAFE, INC.

Luv My Kitty ✍
A truly economical, effective, and convenient all-natural litter made from 100% recycled wood products (pure

sawdust). Available at cat shows or by mail from the manufacturer with free shipping to anywhere in the U.S. It's 2½ times more absorbent than clay, completely odor-free, and safe for you and your cat.

GLOBAL SPECIALTY PET FOODS

Best Breed Organic Cat Litter
Made from plant material, these small green pellets are flushable, compostable, and effective at eliminating cat box odors. More absorbent than clay and lasts longer, too. As of this writing, available only by mail-order.

GRAIN PROCESSING CORP.

World's Best Cat Litter™ ✍
This litter really lives up to its name! These granules made from corn resemble Grape-Nuts™ cereal in size, texture, and consistency. Even the most litter resistant cats adapt easily to World's Best. It clumps perfectly so you can just scoop and flush it away. It is 99% dust free, organic, safe, and because it lasts longer than clay, it's economical too. When using this litter, the cat box is virtually odorless! These folks also make the world's best litter scoop.

HEARTLAND PRODUCTS, INC.

Heartland Wheat™ Litter
Made from 100% whole wheat with active enzymes that eliminate offensive ammonia odors. Scoopable (it forms solid clumps that become harder the longer they sit!) flushable, dust-free, and completely safe.

NATURAL PET LITTERS, INC.

Little Tiger's Natural Cat Litter ✍
An economical natural pine-wood pellet litter that has excellent odor-absorbing qualities, is environmentally friendly, and safe for you and your pets. A portion of the company's profits are donated to organizations that focus on the preservation of tigers and other big cats.

NATURE'S EARTH PRODUCTS, INC.

Feline Pine™ 🐾
Made of compressed, natural-pine wood pellets that naturally neutralize odors. It is 100% dust-free, pure, safe, healthy, economical, flushable, biodegradable, and can even be used as compost or mulch.

PET CARE SYSTEMS, INC.

Swheat Scoop®
Made with wheat and milo (sorghum). Scoopable, flushable, natural, and safe. Available in pet stores and natural foods markets.

City Litter®
Find this great wheat-based litter in your local supermarket's pet food aisle.

Wheat 'N Easy
Available through your veterinarian.

WYSONG CORPORATION

Wysong Litter Lite™
Litter Lite is made from byproducts of the paper-milling industry. These cellulose pellets are biodegradable, com postable, economical, and free of allergenic chemicals.

Note: Some cats may resist change to a new type of litter. When I first tried introducing my cat to pellet litter all at once, he would urinate in his box, but poop behind the futon in my guest room. He soon taught me that the best way to introduce a cat to a change in litter product, is to mix ¼ part new litter with ¾ parts of the old brand. Gradually decrease the amount of old litter until your cat has adjusted to the new litter.

Networking Resources

Write or call the following organizations for information on vegetarianism and related subjects:

American Natural Hygiene Society
12816 Race Track Road
Tampa, FL 33625
813-855-6607

American Vegan Society
Box H
Malaga, NJ 08328
609-694-2887

EarthSave International
600 Distillery Commons, Suite 200
Louisville, KY 40206-1922
502-589-7676

Eating with Conscience Campaign
Humane Society of the United States
700 Professional Drive
Gaithersburg, MD 20879
301-258-3054

Farm Animal Reform Movement (FARM)
Box 30654
Bethesda, MD 20824
301-530-5747

Farm Sanctuary East
P.O. Box 150
Watkins Glen, NY 14891
607-583-2225

Farm Sanctuary West
P.O. Box 1065
Orland, CA 95963
916-865-4617

Friends Vegetarian Society of North America (Quaker)
P.O. Box 53354
Washington, DC 20009

Jewish Vegetarians of North America
6938 Reliance Road
Federalsburg, MD 21632
410-754-5550

North American Vegetarian Society
P.O. Box 72
Dolgeville, NY 13329
518-568-7970

People for the Ethical Treatment of Animals (PETA)
501 Front Street
Norfolk, VA 23570
757-622-1078

Physicians Committee for Responsible Medicine (PCRM)
5100 Wisconsin Ave., Suite 404
Washington, DC 20016
202-686-2210

United Poultry Concerns
P.O. Box 150
Machipongo, VA 23405
757-678-7875

Vegan Action
P.O. Box 4353
Berkeley, CA 94704
510-654-6297

Vegetarian Awareness Network
P.O. Box 321
Knoxville, TN 37901
800-EAT-VEGE

Vegetarian Resource Group
P.O. Box 1463
Baltimore, MD 21203
410-366-VEGE

Vegetarian Union of North America (VUNA)
P.O. Box 9710
Washington, DC 20016
617-625-3790

Vegetarian Resources on the Internet

The following websites provide valuable information on a variety of topics of interest to vegetarians. You can get answers to health questions, download the latest news articles and recipes, find out about exciting vegetarian events, become informed about animal rights issues, learn about the environmental impact of your food choices, and even chat with other vegetarians. Many of these sites will link you to other websites. Once you begin exploring the web, you'll discover many more resources on your own.

Animal Rights Resource Site
http://arrs.envirolink.org

A comprehensive and well-organized source of information about all aspects of animal rights, including a platform for free and open discussion.

EarthSave International
http://www.earthsave.org

EarthSave International is a nonprofit global movement that promotes the benefits of plant-based foods for personal health, a sustainable environment, and a more compassionate world.

Farm Animal Reform Movement (FARM)
http://arrs.envirolink.org/farm

Farm Animal Reform Movement campaigns for the rights of farmed animals, promotes wholesome plant-based eating, and encourages environmental consciousness. Visit this site to learn about FARM's five national programs, including the Great American Meatout.

Farm Sanctuary
http://www.farmsanctuary.org

Farm Sanctuary is dedicated to stopping the exploitation of animals used for food production. Since its inception in 1986, Farm Sanctuary has devoted its resources and time to exposing and ending the cruel practices of the "food animal" industry. This website provides a wide range of information on campaigns to fight animal abuses, news articles, and vegetarianism.

New Veg
http://www.newveg.av.org

Not just for the new or wanna-be vegetarian, NewVeg is a non-profit organization dedicated to smashing myths and delivering the truth regarding human nutrition. This site is for people interested in learning more about a cholesterol-free (vegan) diet with an emphasis on raw foods. NewVeg is also a great entertainment value for all the many dedicated veggie veterans out there in cyberland.

North American Vegetarian Society (NAVS)
http://www.cyberveg.org/navs

NAVS is a nonprofit educational organization dedicated to promoting vegetarianism. At this website you can get info about and register to attend Summerfest, an annual conference presented by the North American Vegetarian Society for the past twenty-four years. At Summerfest you can learn from experts in the fields of health, nutrition, exercise, animal rights, and the environment. It's a wonderful opportunity to meet, socialize, and have fun with others who share similar interests, learn how to prepare delicious vegetarian cuisine with renowned cooking instructors, and eat great tasting, totally vegetarian food.

Notmilk and The Anti-Dairy Coalition
http://www.notmilk.com

A great resource for learning about alternatives to dairy products and insight into what's wrong with milk.

People for the Ethical Treatment of Animals (PETA)
http://www.peta-online.org

PETA's website features Action Alerts that provide timely information on how you can help bring about a more compassionate world through simple, effective, direct actions. The Activist's Library gives visitors access to magazines, factsheets, videos, photos, and other related resources. The Compassionate Living page offers vegetarian recipes, shopping guides, and more daily life ways to help the animals. PETA Kids is a new section of the website with all of the information kids, parents, and educators need to get more involved in animal rights.

Physicians Committee for Responsible Medicine (PCRM)
http://www.sai.com/pcrm

PCRM is a nonprofit organization comprised of doctors and laypersons working together for compassionate and effective medical practice, research and health promotion. This website offers news releases and a guide to private health foundations. The guide identifies which foundations fund animal research and those which do not. PCRM promotes preventive medicine through innovative programs such as The Gold Plan, a program of healthful eating for businesses, hospitals, and schools. The New Four Food Groups is PCRM's innovative proposal for a federal nutrition policy that puts a new priority on health.

The Jewish Vegan Lifestyle
http://www.goodnet.com/~tjvmab

The purpose of The Jewish Vegan Lifestyle is to promote the practice of a vegan lifestyle within the Torah laws, both written and oral. At this website you will find Veggie-Rebbie frequently asked questions and answers, Jewish vegan/vegetarian contacts, a worldwide events calendar, book reviews, kosher food alerts, a guide to kosher vegan and vegetarian restaurants, and personals listings for single Jewish vegans and vegetarians.

Vegan Action
http://www.vegan.org

Vegan Action is a nonprofit grassroots activist organization focused on promoting the vegan diet and lifestyle and inspiring more people to become actively involved in the vegan movement.

Vegan Foundation
http://www.vegan.com

A compilation of timely articles on health, animals, and the environment with links to resources of interest to vegans.

Vegan Outreach
http://www.veganoutreach.org

Vegan Outreach is an international nonprofit organization dedicated to furthering education and understanding in order to bring about fundamental change in our physical well-being, our treatment of others, and our interaction with our environment. VO is working to promote veganism through the widespread distribution of its illustrated booklet, *Why Vegan*. You can read this highly informative pamphlet by visiting their website.

Vegetarian Central
http://www.vegetariancentral.org

The starting point for vegetarian information on the Internet. Currently contains links to over 200 sites.

Vegetarian Pages
http://www.veg.org/veg

Intended to be the definitive guide to what is available on the Internet for vegetarians, vegans, and others.

Vegetarian Resource Group
http://www.vrg.org

Here visitors can play a game and test their nutritional knowledge. You can sign up for VRG's free e-mail newsletter VRG-News and subscribe to the *Vegetarian Journal* online. Also check out VRG's catalog featuring books about vegetarianism, magazines, T-shirts, and bumper stickers.

Vegetarian Society U.K.
http://www.veg.org/veg/Orgs/VegSocUK

Established in 1847, the aim of The Vegetarian Society is to increase the number of vegetarians in order to save animals, benefit human health, and protect the environment and world food resources. The society, a registered charity, is dedicated to fund raising to drive its diverse programs in the areas of campaigning, education, information, and research. Their website is a resource for the new vegetarian, and provides information on health and nutrition, animals and the environment, a recipes index, and the youth pages, devoted specifically to young people interested in vegetarianism.

Vegetarian Union of North America (VUNA)
http://www.ivu.org/vuna

This multi-lingual website is dedicated to promoting a strong, effective, cooperative vegetarian movement throughout North America. VUNA's aim is to supply vegetarian organizations and individuals with information that will help them organize and maintain a strong vegetarian lifestyle.

Veggies Unite!
http://www.vegweb.com

A wonderful resource for vegetarians featuring a chat room, weekly newsletter, a useful grocery list maker and weekly meal planner, book reviews, a recipe directory to over 2,000 vegan recipes, articles, and more.

VegSource
http://www.vegsource.com

Your news, information, and discussion site for all things related to vegetarianism, animals, the environment, and more. Features a variety of message boards, illuminating articles, recipes, and travel information. VegSource also hosts the web pages of many leading vegetarian experts.

World Guide to Vegetarianism
http://catless.ncl.ac.uk/veg/Guide

A massive listing of vegetarian and vegetarian-friendly restaurants, stores, organizations, and services.

Glossary

AMARANTH
An ancient Aztec grain, ranging in color from purple to yellow. High in fiber, and rich in calcium, iron, and phosphorus. Amaranth is also gluten-free.

AMAZAKE
A refreshing Japanese drink made from organic whole-grain brown rice. Cultured rice (called koji) is added to the cooled whole grain allowing a natural sweetness to develop creating a flavorful nectar-like beverage.

BABAGANOUSH
Middle Eastern purée of eggplant, sesame seed paste, olive oil, lemon juice, and garlic that is served as a spread or dip.

BASMATI RICE
An East Indian specialty of long-grain rice that is aged for a year to enhance its flavor. It has a chewy texture and a nutty taste.

BURRITO
From Mexican cookery, a folded and rolled flour tortilla stuffed with various savory fillings. Vegetarian burritos may be filled with shredded or chopped vegetables, cheese, or beans.

CHAI
It's the word for tea in many parts of the world, particularly southern Asia. Chai from India is a spiced milk tea that is blended with a combination of exotic spices and a sweetener. The spices used vary from region to region, but the most common are cardamom, cinnamon, ginger, cloves, and pepper. Indian chai produces a warming, soothing effect, acts as a natural digestive aid and gives one a wonderful sense of well-being.

CHAPATI
An unleavened round, flat bread from India, usually made from a simple mixture of whole-wheat flour and water.

Chicory
A perennial plant often cultivated for its root, which when roasted and ground is used as a substitute or additive to coffee.

Chipotle Chile
Jalapeño chile with a sweet, smoky flavor.

Chorizo
Used in both Mexican and Spanish cooking, chorizo is a highly seasoned, coarsely ground sausage flavored with garlic, chili powder, and other spices. Before cooking chorizo, the casing is removed and the sausage is crumbled. Vegetarian chorizo may be added to a variety of dishes including soups, stews, and scrambled tofu.

Chutney
A spicy condiment from India made with fruit, vinegar, sugar, and spices. Chutney is the traditional accompaniment to curried dishes. It can range in spiciness from mild to hot.

Couscous
From the Middle East, couscous is a cooked, bulgur-type grain made from granular semolina. Often eaten as a side dish, salad, or sometimes sweetened for a dessert.

Enchilada
A Mexican dish made by rolling a softened corn tortilla around a vegetable filling. Enchiladas are often topped with cheese.

Falafel
A Middle Eastern specialty, falafel are small, deep-fried patties or balls made of spiced, ground chickpeas. They are usually stuffed inside pita bread with shredded lettuce, tomatoes, and tahini sauce to create a tasty sandwich.

Gelatin
A tasteless and colorless thickening agent, derived from animal bones, cartilage, tendons, hooves, and other tissue used to make fruity gel-like desserts. Vegetarian gelatin alternatives are readily available (see kosher gelatin on the following page).

HEMP SEED
From the plant cannabis sativa, hemp seed is a highly nutritious source of protein and essential fatty acids that rivals the soybean for its nutritional value. Hemp seeds have a nutty taste and are used to make a variety of food products including hempeh burgers.

HUMMUS
A thick Middle Eastern sauce made from mashed chickpeas, lemon juice, garlic, and olive oil. It's served as a sauce or as a dip with pieces of pita bread.

JALAPEÑO CHILI
Smooth, dark-green chile peppers with extremely hot seeds and stems.

KASHA
From Eastern European cookery, kasha is a cooked dish prepared from hulled and crushed grain that is then roasted. It can be made of millet or oats, but in America, kasha is generally made from buckwheat groats. It is often eaten as a side dish or used as a filling for knishes.

KNISH
A Jewish pastry consisting of a piece of dough wrapped around a filling of mashed potatoes, vegetables, kasha, or cheese. Knishes can be served as a side dish or appetizer. Dessert knishes can be made with a sweet, fruity filling.

KOSHER GELATIN
Plant-derived gelatins made from agar-agar, carageenan, (a dried seaweed product) or locust bean gum. Kosher gelatins are available in plain or fruit flavors.

MASA
Masa is the traditional dough used to make corn tortillas and tamales. It is made with sun- or fire-dried corn kernels that have been cooked, soaked in lime water, and then ground into meal.

MILLET
A small, round, golden grain that is prepared much like rice and is rich in protein. It is often eaten as a hot cereal or mixed with seasonings and served as a side dish.

MISO
A staple in Japanese cooking, miso is a thick, spreadable, salty paste made from cooked, aged soybeans, barley, or rice. It's used in flavoring soup bases, sauces, dips, salad dressings, and main dishes.

MOLE
This rich, flavorful sauce is a Mexican specialty. Made up of a smooth, cooked mixture of onions, garlic, several varieties of chiles, herbs, spices, and ground sesame or pumpkin seeds. Some variations of mole also contain a small amount of Mexican chocolate that contributes richness to the sauce without adding too much sweetness.

NAAN
An East Indian, flattened, round white-flour bread that is lightly leavened. It is traditionally baked in a tandoor (brick and clay) oven.

PÂTÉ
Vegetarian pâté is made from a finely ground or chunky mixture of vegetables, mushrooms, nuts, or seeds. A pâté can be satiny-smooth and spreadable, or like country pâté, coarsely textured. Pâtés are usually served as an appetizer along with crackers or small pieces of bread.

PIEROGI
A Polish specialty, pierogies are half moon-shaped noodle dumplings filled with a minced mixture of potatoes, cheese, and spices.

RAMEN
A Japanese dish of noodles and vegetables in a delicately seasoned broth.

SAMOSA
From India, samosas are fried, triangular pastries stuffed with a savory vegetable mixture and often served as an appetizer with chutney.

SEITAN
Also called wheat meat, seitan is a protein-rich food made from wheat gluten. It has a firm, chewy texture making it an ideal

substitute for meat (especially chicken). Neutral in flavor, seitan easily picks up the flavors of the sauces, spices, and other foods with which it is cooked.

SHOYU
Japanese for soy sauce.

SOY SAUCE
A staple in Asian cooking, soy sauce is a dark, salty sauce made by fermenting boiled soybeans and roasted wheat or barley. It is used to flavor soups, rice dishes, marinades, and vegetables, and as a table condiment as well.

TAHINI
A thick, smooth paste made of ground sesame seeds from the Middle East.

TAMALE
A Mexican dish made of various fillings coated with a masa dough and then wrapped in a softened corn husk. The tamale is steamed until the dough is cooked through and the corn husk is peeled back before the tamale is eaten. Tamales can be savory (filled with a mixture of mashed vegetables), or sweet (stuffed with fruit or other dessert filling).

TAMARIND
The fruit of a tall shade tree native to Asia and northern Africa and widely grown in India. Large pods contain small seeds and a sour-sweet pulp that when dried, becomes extremely sour. Tamarind pulp concentrate is popular as a flavoring in East Indian cuisine and is used to season foods such as chutneys and curry dishes.

TEMPEH
An Indonesian soy food made from cultured soybeans that are then pressed into bar form. Tempeh is high in protein and chewy in texture, making it a wonderful meat substitute.

TERRINE
A pâté that has been cooked in a container called a terrine or any other similar type of mold.

TOFU
Popular throughout the Orient, tofu is a white curd made by washing, soaking, grinding, and boiling soybeans, adding coagulant, and then pressing the substance into a solid form. It's available in different textures such as soft, silken, hard, firm, and extra firm. When cooked with sauces and seasonings, tofu easily takes on their flavors.

TORTILLA
The staple bread of Mexico, the tortilla is an unleavened, round, and flat bread resembling a very thin pancake. It can be made from corn flour (masa) or wheat flour, and is baked on a griddle. Tortillas are used for making burritos, enchiladas, tacos, and a variety of other dishes.

TOSTADT
A crisply baked tortilla covered with a variety of toppings such as chopped vegetables, refried beans, cheese, lettuce, tomatoes, sour cream, and guacamole.

TRITICALE
An extremely nutritious hybrid of wheat and rye with a nutty-sweet flavor.

TVP
Textured Vegetable Protein (or TVP) is concentrated soy protein. It can be used to extend or replace meat in chili, meatballs, casseroles, and an endless variety of dishes. It is the base for many of the ground-meat substitutes available.

VINAIGRETTE
A tart sauce of oil, vinegar, and seasonings, usually used as a salad dressing.

YUBA
A bean curd "skin" that forms on soy milk when it is heated. This very delicate skin is carefully removed and then dried in sheets or folded into sticks. Yuba sheets are used to wrap other foods that can be braised, deep-fried, or steamed.

Suggested Reading

Akers, Keith A., *A Vegetarian Sourcebook: The Nutrition, Ecology, and Ethics of a Natural Foods Diet*, Vegetarian Press, 1993.

Attwood, Charles, R., M.D., *Dr. Attwood's Low-Fat Prescription for Kids*, Viking, 1995.

——, *A Vegetarian Doctor Speaks Out*, Hohm Press, 1998.

Barnard, Neal, M.D., *Eat Right, Live Longer*, Crown, 1995.

——, *Food for Life: How the New Four Food Groups Can Save Your Life*, Harmony Books, 1993.

——, *Foods that Fight Pain*, Harmony Books, 1998.

——, *The Power of Your Plate*, Book Publishing Company, 1990.

Berry, Rynn, *Food for the Gods: Vegetarianism & the World's Religions*, Pythagorean Publishers, 1998.

Bonvie, Linda, Bonvie, Bill, and Gates, Donna, *The Stevia Story: A Tale of Incredible Sweetness & Intrigue*, B.E.D. Publications, 1997.

Cohen, Robert, *Milk: The Deadly Poison*, Argus Publishing, 1998.

Eisnitz, Gail A., *Slaughterhouse*, Prometheus Books, 1997.

Fox, Michael W., D.V.M., *Agricide*, Shocken Books, 1986.

——, *Eating with Conscience: The Bioethics of Food*, NewSage Press, 1997.

Kalechovsky, Roberta, Ph.D.,*Vegetarian Judaism: A Guide for Everyone*, Micah Publications, 1998.

Klaper, Michael, M.D., *Pregnancy, Childbirth, and the Vegan Diet*, Gentle World, 1988.

——, *Vegan Nutrition: Pure and Simple*, Gentle World, 1987.

Kradjian, Robert, *Save Yourself from Breast Cancer*, Berkeley Publishing Group, 1994.

Lyman, Howard F., *Mad Cowboy: Plain Truth from the Cattle Rancher Who Won't Eat Meat*, Scribner, 1998.

Marcus, Erik, *Vegan: The New Ethics of Eating*, McBooks Press, 1998.

Martin, Ann N., *Foods Pets Die For: Shocking Facts about Pet Food*, NewSage Press, 1997.

Mason, Jim, and Singer, Peter, *Animal Factories*, Harmony

Books, 1980.

McDougall, John A., M.D., *McDougall's Medicine: A Challenging Second Opinion*, New Century Publishers, 1985.

McDougall, John A., M.D., and McDougall, Mary, *The McDougall Program: 12 Days to Dynamic Health*, Penguin Books, 1990.

Moran, Victoria, *The Love-Powered Diet*, New World Library, 1992.

Oski, Frank, M.D., *Don't Drink Your Milk!*, Teach Services, 1983.

Peden, James, *Vegetarian Cats and Dogs*, Harbingers of a New Age, 1995.

Reinhardt, Mark Warren, *The Perfectly Contented Meat-Eater's Guide to Vegetarianism*, Continuum, 1998.

Rifkin, Jeremy, *Beyond Beef: The Rise and Fall of the Cattle Culture*, Dutton Books, 1992.

Robbins, John, *Diet for a New America*, Stillpoint Publishing, 1987.

Cookbooks

Costigan, Fran, *You Won't Believe these are Healthy Desserts*, For Goodness Cakes, 1998.

DePuydt, Rita, *Baking with Stevia*, Sun Coast Enterprises, 1997.

Diamond, Marilyn, *The American Vegetarian Cookbook*, Random House, 1990.

Hutchins, Imar, *Delights of the Garden: Vegetarian Cuisine Prepared without Heat*, Doubleday, 1994.

Nishimoto, Miyoko, *The Now and Zen Epicure*, Book Publishing Company, 1991.

Newkirk, Ingrid, *The Compassionate Cook*, Warner Books, 1993.

Raymond, Jennifer, *Fat Free & Easy: Great Meals in Minutes*, Book Publishing Company, 1997.

——, *The Peaceful Palate*, Heart & Soul Publications, 1992.

Soria, Cherie, *Angel Foods*, Heartstar Productions, 1996.

Stepaniak, Joanne, *The Uncheese Cookbook*, Book Publishing Company, 1994.

——, *Vegan Vittles*, Book Publishing Company, 1996.

Wasserman, Debra, *Conveniently Vegan*, Vegetarian Resource Group, 1997.

Wasserman, Debra, and Stahler, Charles, *Meatless Meals for Working People*, Vegetarian Resource Group, 1991.

Index of Suppliers

Companies that sell products through mail-order are highlighted with an asterisk(*).

A & A Amazing Foods, Inc.
PO Box 3927
Citrus Heights, CA 95611
800-275-1437

Adambra Imports, Inc.
585 Meserole St.
Brooklyn, NY 11237
718-628-9700

* **Adeline's Gourmet Foods**
5036 Venice Blvd.
Los Angeles, CA 90019
888-773-FOOD

* **Alcala Enterprises**
12824 Hadley St. #106
Whittier, CA 90601
562-945-1683

Allied Old English, Inc.
100 Markley St.
Port Reading, NJ 07064
800-225-0122

* **Allison's Cookies**
11814 105th SW, Suite A
Vashon, WA 98070
206-567-5292

AlpineAir Foods
13321 Grass Valley Ave.
Grass Valley, CA 95959
800-322-6325

Alpursa
PO Box 25846
Salt Lake City, UT 84125
801-965-8428

Alternative Baking
Company, Inc.
4865 Pasadena Ave., Suite 1
Sacramento, CA 95841
888-488-9725

Amberwave Foods
201 Ann St.
Oakmont, PA 15139
800-875-3040

American Health Kennels
4351 NE 11th Ave.
Pompano Beach, FL 33064
800-940-DOGS

American Natural Snacks
PO Box 1067
St. Augustine, FL 32085
800-238-3947

American Nutrition
PO Box 1405
Ogden, UT 84402
800-257-4530

* **American Spoon Foods, Inc.**
PO Box 566
Petosky, MI 49770
888-735-6700

Amy's Kitchen Inc.
PO Box 449
Petaluma, CA 94953
707-762-6194

Arrowhead Mills, Inc.
PO Box 2059
Hereford, TX 79045
800-749-0730

Artisan Foods
407 N. Nopal St.
Santa Barbara, CA 93103
805-884-0337

* Asparagus Enterprises, Inc.
PO Box 900
DeWitt, MI 48820
888-669-4250

Aspen Pet Products, Inc.
11701 E. 53rd Ave.
Denver, CO 80239
303-375-1001

* Backpacker's Pantry
6350 Gunpark Dr.
Boulder, CO 80301
800-253-8283

Barbara's Bakery, Inc.
3900 Cypress Dr.
Petaluma, CA 94954
707-765-2273

Ben & Jerry's Homemade, Inc.
Rt. 100
Waterbury, VT 05676
802-651-9600

* Big Sur Coast Foods
HC67, Box 1388
Big Sur, CA 93920
408-667-2217

Bioforce of America Ltd.
PO Box 507
Kinderhook, NY 12106
800-645-9135

* Blanchard & Blanchard Ltd.
PO Box 1080
Norwich, VT 05055
800-334-0268

Bliss' San Francisco
19 Bowman Ct.
San Francisco, CA 94124
415-285-9709

* Blossom Products Co.
6900 E. Camelback Rd. #700
Scottsdale, AZ 85251
602-947-7677

Blue Diamond Growers
PO Box 1768
Sacramento, CA 95812
916-442-0771

Blue Sky Natural Foods
510 Don Gaspar
Santa Fe, NM 87501
505-986-8777

Boca Burger Company
1660 NE 12th Terrace
Ft. Lauderdale, FL 33305
954-524-4171

* Body Ecology
1266 W. Paces Ferry Rd.,
Suite 505
Atlanta, GA 30327
800-4-STEVIA

* Boss Bars
PO Box 517
Patagonia, AZ 85624
520-394-2370
For mail orders call
Morrill's New Directions
at: 800-368-5057

Boulder Bar Endurance, Inc.
PO Box 712083
San Diego, CA 92171
619-279-8463

* Brunzi's Best, Inc.
RR1 Box 63
Garrison, NY 10524
914-734-4490

* BT Trading Company
PO Box 852742
Richardson, TX 75085
972-437-4151

Bush Brothers & Company
PO Box 52330, Dept. C
Knoxville, TN 37950
423-588-7685

California Natural Products
PO Box 1219
Lathrop, CA 95330
209-858-2525

* Cary Randall's
PO Box 363
Highlands, NJ 07732
888-88-NOFAT

Cascadian Farm
719 Metcalf St.
Sedro-Woolley, WA 98284
800-624-4123

Cedarlane Natural Foods, Inc.
1864 E. 22nd St.
Los Angeles, CA 90058
800-826-3322

Celentano
225 Bloomfield Ave.
Verona, NJ 07044
201-239-8444

Cemac Foods Corp.
1821 E. Sedgley Ave.
Philadelphia, PA 19124
800-724-0179

* Chocolate Decadence
1050-D Bethel Dr.
Eugene, OR 97402
800-324-5018

* Chocolate Emporium
14439 Cedar Rd.
South Euclid, OH 44121
888-CHOCLAT

Cloud Nine Inc.
300 Observer Hwy., Third Fl.
Hoboken, NJ 07030
201-216-0382

* Cowboy Caviar
1552 Beach St., Suite G
Emeryville, CA 94608
510-594-8051

* Coyote Cocina
1590 San Mateo Lane
Santa Fe, NM 87505
800-866-HOWL

* D'Artagnan, Inc.
399-419 St. Paul Ave.
Jersey City, NJ 07306
800-327-8246

Dandy Doggie
15 Woodland Ave., Suite E
San Rafael, CA 94901
888-236-4568

* Della Terra, Inc.
5438 Rt. 14
Dundee, NY 14837
888-DT FOODS

Deep Foods, Inc.
1090 Springfield Rd.
Union, NJ 07083
800-468-6499

Del Sol Food Co., Inc.
PO Box 2243
Brenham, TX 77834
409-836-5978

Devansoy Farms, Inc.
PO Box 885
Carroll, IA 51401
800-747-8605

Discovery Foods
2395 American Ave.
Hayward, CA 94545
510-293-1838

Dolphin Natural Chocolates
1975 Woodview Ave.
Cambria, CA 93428
800-2-DOLPHIN

Double Rainbow
Gourmet Ice Creams, Inc.
275 South Van Ness Ave.
San Francisco, CA 94103
800-489-3580

* Dr. McDougall's Right Foods
101 Utah Ave.
So. San Francisco, CA 94080
415-635-6000

Dreyer's Grand Ice Cream
5929 College Ave.
Oakland, CA 94618
800-888-3442

* Earthsafe, Inc.
PO Box 424
Lavonia, GA 30553
800-200-0140

* Earth/Sun Farm
PO Box 99
Dixon, NM 87527
505-579-4246

Eden Foods, Inc.
701 Tecumseh Rd.
Clinton, MI 49236
800-248-0320

Edward & Sons Trading
Co., Inc.
PO Box 1326
Carpinteria, CA 93014
805-684-8500

El Burrito Mexican Food Co.
PO Box 90125
Industry, CA 91715
800-933-7828

* Ener-G Foods, Inc.
PO Box 84487
Seattle, WA 98124
800-331-5222

* Equinox International
Phone orders for Equi-Milk
Item #3115
Reference #1160959
800-519-7777

* Essence of India
PO Box 24568
Minneapolis, MN 55424
612-935-5999

Eskimo Pie Corp.
901 Moorefield Park Dr.
Richmond, VA 23236
804-560-8400

* Evolution Pet Foods
287 E. 6th. St., Suite 270
St. Paul, MN 55101
651-228-0632

Fantastic Foods Inc.
1250 N. McDowell Blvd.
Petaluma, CA 94954
707-778-7801

First Light Foods
60 E. Elm St.
Chicago, IL 60611
800-555-4332

* **Flo's Delicious Food**
1516 Buena Vista SE
Albuquerque, NM 87106
505-232-0100

Florida Crystals, Inc.
50 Cocoanut Row #215
Palm Beach, FL 33480
561-822-5900

Follow Your Heart
7848 Alabama Ave.
Canoga Park, CA 91304
818-347-9946

Food From The 'Hood
c/o Crenshaw High School
5010 11th Ave.
Los Angeles, CA 90043
213-295-4842

Frankly Natural Bakers
7740 Formula Pl.
San Diego, CA 92126
619-274-4000

* **Fresh Tofu, Inc.**
PO Box 1125
Easton, PA 18044
610-258-0883

Fruitsource Associates
1803 Mission St. #404
Santa Cruz, CA 95060
831-457-1196

Fuller Life, Inc.
1628 Robert C. Jackson Dr.
Maryville, TN 37801
800-227-2320

Gabila and Sons
Manufacturing, Inc.
120 S. 8th St.
Brooklyn, NY 11211
718-387-0750

Galaxy Foods Co.
2441 Viscount Row
Orlando, FL 32809
407-855-5500

Garden of Eatin' Inc.
5300 Santa Monica Blvd.
Los Angeles, CA 90029
213-462-5406

Gardenburger, Inc.
1411 SW Morrison St.,
Suite 400
Portland, OR 97205
800-636-0109

Garlic Valley Farms
624 Roberta Ave.
Glendale, CA 91201
800-424-7990

* **Geetha's Gourmet Products**
1589 Imperial Ridge
Las Cruces, NM 88011
800-274-0475

Ghirardelli Chocolate Company
1111 139th Ave.
San Leandro, CA 94578
800-877-9338

Glacier Gourmet, Inc.
25437 Rye Canyon Rd.
Santa Clarita, CA 91355
800-257-4947

* **Global Specialty Pet Foods**
15029 US 224 E
Findlay, OH 45840
800-500-5999

Gloria's Kitchen
PO Box 2071
Burlingame, CA 94011
650-579-0638

Glorybee Foods
120 N. Seneca
Eugene, OR 97402
541-689-0913

Golden Valley Foods
7450 Metro Blvd.
Edina, MN 55439
612-835-6900

Goldwater's Foods of Arizona
PO Box 9846
Scottsdale, AZ 85252
800-488-4932

* **Gourmet Tamales**
2588 El Camino Real D-228
Carlsbad, CA 92008
760-729-0387

* **Grain Processing Corp.**
1600 Oregon St.
Muskateen, IA 52761
877-FOR-WBCL

Grainaissance, Inc.
1580 62nd St.
Emeryville, CA 94608
800-GRAIN-97

Green Options, Inc.
2262 Palou Ave.
San Francisco, CA 94124
888-GREEN-OP

Greene's Farm
5590 High St.
Denver, CO 80216
800-748-2972

Guiltless Gourmet, Inc.
3709 Promontory Point Dr.
#131
Austin, TX 78744
512-443-4373

The Hain Food Group, Inc.
50 Charles Lindbergh Blvd.
Uniondale, NY 11553
800-434-HAIN

* **Harbingers of a New Age**
717 E. Missoula Ave.
Troy, Montana 59935
800-884-6262

* **Harvest Direct, Inc.**
PO Box 988
Knoxville, TN 37901
800-835-2867

* **Hawaiian Fruit Specialties Ltd.**
PO Box 637
Kalaheo, Kauai, HI 96741
808-828-1761

Health is Wealth Inc.
Sykes Lane
Williamstown, NJ 08094
609-728-1998

Health Trip Foods, Inc.
50 Beharrell St.
Concord, MA 01742
978-287-0200

Health Valley Foods
16100 Foothill Blvd.
Irwindale, CA 91706
800-423-4846

Heartland Products, Inc.
PO Box 777
Valley City, ND 58072
800-437-4780

* Hempzels/A Division of
No Problem, Inc.
PO Box 13
New Holland, PA 17557
800-USE-HEMP

HKS Marketing, Ltd.
420 Kent St.
Brooklyn, NY 11211
718-384-2400

* Holy Chipotle
369 Montezuma #451
Santa Fe, NM 87501
800-992-HOLY

Hormel Foods Corporation
1 Hormel Place
Austin, MN 55912
800-523-4635

Hot Mama's Ravioli, Etc.
1485 Gericke Rd.
Petaluma, CA 94952
707-778-3441

The Hot Tomato Kitchens, Inc.
Route 31, Box 197K
Santa Fe, NM 87505
888-6-TOMATO

Howler Products
2685 Elizabeth Court
Sebastopol, CA 95472
800-HOWLERS

Hungry Sultan Mediterranean
Gourmet
4040 Civic Center Drive,
Suite 200
San Rafael, CA 94903
888-2-SULTAN

Hunt-Wesson, Inc.
PO Box 4800
Fullerton, CA 92634
800-633-0112

I-D Foods Corporation
2585 Skymark
Mississauga, Ontario
L4W 4L5 Canada
888-ID-FOODS

Imagine Foods, Inc.
350 Cambridge Ave., Suite #350
Palo Alto, CA 94306
415-327-1444

Integrated Brands Inc.
4175 Veterans Hwy.
Ronkonkoma, NY 11779
800-423-2763

* International Business
Trade, Inc.
4624 W. Esplanade,
Suite 101
Metairie, LA 70006
504-457-2047

International ProSoya Corp.
312-19292 60th Ave.
Surrey, BC V3S 8E5 Canada
604-532-8030

Internatural Foods, Inc.
15 Prospect St.
Paramus, NJ 07652
201-262-4830

Internova Inc.
1071, St-Aimé, PO Box 727
St-Lambert de Levis, Québec,
G0S 2W0 Canada
800-993-6455

J&J Snack Foods Corp.
5353 Downey Rd.
Vernon, CA 90058
213-581-0171

Jacqui's Gourmet Cookies, Etc.
664A Freeman Ln., Suite 204
Grass Valley, CA 95949
800-310-0107

* **The Just Tomatoes Company**
PO Box 807
Westley, CA 95387
800-537-1985

Kali's Sportnaturals, Inc.
1610 Fifth St.
Berkeley, CA 94710
800-884-KALI

Knudsen & Sons, Inc.
PO Box 369
Chico, CA 95927
530-899-5010

Kraft General Foods, Inc.
250 North St., Box PC7
White Plains, NY 10625
800-432-6333

Lady J Inc.
PO Box 1307
Menlo Park, CA 94025
650-329-0588

* **Lenny & Larry's**
4935 McConnell Ave., Unit 13
Los Angeles, CA 90066
800-LENNY-LARRY

Liberty Richter Inc.
400 Lyster Ave.
Saddle Brook, NJ 07663
800-631-3650

Lightlife Foods, Inc.
153 Industrial Blvd.
Turners Falls, MA 01376
800-274-6001

Lima
PO Box 2205
Placerville, CA 95667
888-400-LIMA

Little Bear Organic Foods
1065 E. Walnut St.
Carson, CA 90746
800-769-6455

Lucky Food Co.
7911 NE 33rd St., Suite 320
Portland, OR 97211
503-287-3801

* **Lumen Foods**
409 Scott St.
Lake Charles, LA 70601
800-256-2253

* **Maharishi Ayur-Ved Products
International, Inc.**
PO Box 49667
Colorado Springs, CO 80949
800-255-8332

Maranatha Natural Foods
PO Box 1046
Ashland, OR 97520
541-488-2747

Martin Brothers
PO Box 1686
Austin, TX 78767
512-478-4434

* McCutcheon Apple
  Products, Inc.
  PO Box 243
  Frederick, MD 21705
  800-875-3451

* Mental Processes, Inc.
  1075 Zonolite Rd.
  Atlanta, GA 30306
  800-431-4018

* Milagro Country Foods
  1800 Central Ave. SE
  Albuquerque, NM 87106
  800-MILAGRO

* Modern Products Inc.
  PO Box 09398
  Milwaukee, WI 53209
  414-352-3333

  Morinaga Nutritional
  Foods, Inc.
  2050 W. 190th St., Suite 110
  Torrance, CA 90504
  800-NOW-TOFU

  Mother Nature's Goodies, Inc.
  13378 California St.
  Yucaipa, CA 92399
  909-795-6018

  Mrs. Denson's Cookie
  Company, Inc.
  120 Brush St.
  Ukiah, CA 95482
  707-462-2272

  Mrs. Malibu Foods, Inc.
  23852 PCH, Suite 372
  Malibu, CA 90265
  888-MRS-MALIBU

Mudpie Frozen Foods
2549 Lyndale Ave. South
Minneapolis, MN 55405
612-870-4888

* Muscle Muffins
  3-146th Ave. SE
  Bellevue, WA 98007
  425-641-2106

Nana's Cookie Company
4901 Morena Blvd. #403
San Diego, CA 92117
619-273-5775

Nasoya Foods, Inc.
1 New England Way
Ayer, MA 01432
800-229-TOFU

Natural Feast Corp.
435 Coggeshall St.
New Bedford, MA 02746
508-984-4230

Natural Life, Inc.
PO Box 20492
Floral Park, NY 11002
718-433-4552

Natural Life Pet Products, Inc.
PO Box 943
Frontenac, KS 66763
800-367-2391

Natural Ovens of Manitowoc
Wisconsin
PO Box 730
Manitowoc, WI 54221
800-558-3535

Natural Pet Litters, Inc.
125 Church St., Suite 315
Marietta, GA 30060
770-919-9150

* Nature's Animals, Inc.
628 Waverly Ave.
Mamaroneck, NY 10543
800-DOG-BONE

Nature's Earth Products, Inc.
510 Business Parkway
Royal Palm Beach, FL 33411
800-749-PINE

Nature's Hilights
PO Box 3526
Chico, CA 95927
800-313-6454

Nature's Recipe Pet Foods
341 Bonnie Circle
Corona, CA 91720
800-843-4008

New Morn, Inc.
42 Davis Rd.
Acton, MA 01720
978-263-1201

Newman's Own
246 Post Rd. East
Westport, CT 06880
800-272-0257

Newman's Own Organics
PO Box 2098
Aptos, CA 95001
408-685-2866

Newmarket Foods, Inc.
2210 Pine View Way
Petaluma, CA 94954
707-579-8440

Nile Spice Foods
Box 20581
Seattle, WA 98102
800-265-6453

* Northern Lights Hemp Co.
Box 591
Tolino, BC, V0R 2Z0 Canada
800-880-3699

Northern Soy, Inc.
545 West Ave.
Rochester, NY 14611
716-235-8970

Now & Zen, Inc.
665 22nd St.
San Francisco, CA 94107
800-335-1959

Now Foods
395 S. Glen Ellyn Rd.
Bloomingdale, IL 60108
800-999-8069

* NuNaturals
PO Box 644
Eugene, OR 97440
800-753-HERB

Nylabone Products/TFH
Publications
PO Box 27
Neptune, NJ 07754
800-631-2188

Odwalla, Inc.
120 Stone Pine Rd.
Half Moon Bay, CA 94019
800-ODWALLA

* Only Natural, Inc.
31 Saratoga Blvd.
Island Park, NY 11558
800-866-2887

* Orean's Express, Inc.
817 N. Lake Ave.
Pasadena, CA 91104
818-794-0861

Oregon Chai
725 SE Ninth Ave., Suite T
Portland, OR 97214
888-874-CHAI

P.J. Lisac & Associates, Inc.
9001 SE Lawnfield Rd.
Clackamas, OR 97015
503-652-1988

Pacific Foods of Oregon, Inc.
19480 SW 97th Ave.
Tualatin, OR 97062
503-692-9666

* Papaya John's
PO Box 441
Paia, HI 96779
888-972-7292

The Peaceworks, Inc.
PO Box 1587
New York, NY 10016
800-PEACE-21

Pet Care Systems, Inc.
Box 1529
Detroit Lakes, MN 56502
800-SWHEATS

* PetGuard, Inc.
PO Box 728
Orange Park, FL 32067
800-874-3221
in FL: 800-331-7527

Philchic, Inc.
830 W. Williamson Ave.
Fullerton, CA 92832
714-680-9706

The Pillsbury Company
2866 Pillsbury Center
Minneapolis, MN 55402
800-998-9996 (For Green Giant)

* Poiret International
4100 N. Powerline Rd.,
Suite M-1
Pompano Beach, FL 33073
954-917-8783

Preferred Brands, Inc.
1445 E. Putnam Ave.
Old Greenwich, CT 06878
203-698-4040

Progresso Quality Foods
Company
PO Box 555
Vineland, NJ 08360
800-200-9377

* Purr-Fect Growlings
PO Box 90275
Los Angeles, CA 90009
213-751-3613

Quong Hop & Co.
161 Beacon St.
So. San Francisco, CA 94080
650-873-4444

R.F. Bakery International, Inc.
8101 Orion #6
Van Nuys, CA 91406
800-543-2555

The Rainforest Company
141 Millwell Dr.
St. Louis, MO 63043
800-927-2695

Rapunzel Pure Organics
122 Smith Rd. Ext.
Kinderhook, NY 12106
800-207-2814

Rella Good Cheese Co.
(formerly Sharon's Finest)
Box 5020
Santa Rosa, CA 95402
800-656-9669

* RGE, Inc.
PO Box 23388
Santa Fe, NM 87502
800-838-0773

* Road's End Organics, Inc.
PO Box 104
Underhill Center, VT 05490
877-CHREESE

* Robert's American Gourmet
PO Box 67
Roslyn Heights, NY 11576
800-626-7557

* Robusto Kitchens
PO Box 7061
Corte Madera, CA 94976
415-457-5156

Ruthies Foods
PO Box 1029
Fallbrook, CA 92088
800-RUTHIES

* Saguaro Food Products
860 E. 46th St.
Tucson, AZ 85713
520-884-8049

Sahara Natural Foods, Inc.
PO Box 11844
Berkeley, CA 94704
510-352-5111

Santa Cruz Fine Foods/Division
of R.W. Garcia Co., Inc.
PO Box 8290
San Jose, CA 95155
408-287-4616

Scenario, International Co.
PO Box 24177
Los Angeles, CA 90024
800-400-7772

Seenergy Foods Ltd.
121 Jevlan Dr., Woodbridge
Ontario L4L 8A8 Canada
800-609-7674

* Season's Harvest
52 Broadway
Somerville, MA 02145
800-879-7403

ShariAnn's Organics, Inc.
PO Box 534
Dexter, MI 48130
734-426-0989

Simply Delicious, Inc.
8411 Hwy. NC 86
Cedar Grove, NC 27231
919-732-5294

Soyco Foods/A Division of
Galaxy Foods
2441 Viscount Flow
Orlando, FL 32809
800-441-9419

The SoyNut Butter Co.
102 N. Cook St.
Barrington, IL 60010
800-288-1012

Spectrum Naturals, Inc.
133 Copeland St.
Petaluma, CA 94952
707-778-8900

* The Spice of Life Co.
15445 Ventura Blvd., Suite 115
Sherman Oaks, CA 91403
800-256-2253

Springfield Creamery
29440 Airport Rd.
Eugene, OR 97402
541-689-2911

St. Amour
12112 Beach Blvd.
Stanton, CA 90680
714-903-5366

* **Stevita Company, Inc.**
7650 US Highway 287, #100
Arlington, TX 76001
888-STEVITA

Sun Foods Ltd.
115 McCormack St.
Toronto, Ontario
M6N 1X8 Canada
416-766-8214

* **Sundance Country Farm**
PO Box 2429
Valley Center, CA 92082
888-269-9888

* **Sundance Roasting**
Company, Inc.
PO Box 1886
Sandpoint, ID 83864
208-265-2445

* **Sundance Sweets**
360 Hoover Rd.
Soquel, CA 95073
800-908-0802

Sunspire
2114 Adams Ave.
San Leandro, CA 94577
510-569-9731

The Tamarind Tree, Ltd.
(Annie's Homegrown, Inc.)
395 Main St.
Wakefield, MA 01880
800-HFC-TREE

Taj Gourmet Foods
190 Fountain St.
Framingham, MA 01702
508-875-6212

* **Teeccino Caffé, Inc.**
1720 Las Canoas Rd.
Santa Barbara, CA 93105
800-498-3434

Timber Crest Farms
4791 Dry Creek Rd.
Healdsburg, CA 95448
707-433-8251

Tofutti Brands, Inc.
50 Jackson Dr.
Cranford, NJ 07016
908-272-2400

Tradition Foods Inc.
4710 Woodman Ave.
Sherman Oaks, CA 91423
818-783-8838

Tree of Life, Inc.
PO Box 410
St. Augustine, FL 32085
904-824-4699

Tumaro's Homestyle Kitchens
5300 Santa Monica Blvd.
Los Angeles, CA 90029
213-464-6317

* **Turtle Island Foods**
PO Box 176
Hood River, OR 97031
888-TOFURKY

Turtle Mountain, Inc.
PO Box 70
Junction City, OR 97448
541-998-6778

United Specialty Foods
PO Box 41279
Nashville, TN 37204
888-574-LIFE

VeggieLand
222 New Rd.
Parsippany, NJ 07054
888-808-5540

Vitasoy, Inc.
400 Oyster Point Blvd., Suite 201
S. San Francisco, CA 94080
800-VITASOY

* **Wax Orchards Inc.**
22744 Wax Orchards Rd.
Vashon, WA 98070
800-634-6132

Westbrae Natural Foods
PO Box 48006
Gardena, CA 90248
800-SOY-MILK

Western Commerce Corp.
PO Box 90190
City of Industry, CA 91715
626-333-5225

White Wave, Inc.
6123 Arapahoe
Boulder, CO 80303
303-443-3470

Wholesome Foods
PO Box 2860
Daytona Beach, FL 32120
800-680-1896

Wildwood Natural Foods
135 Bolinas Rd.
Fairfax, CA 94930
800-499-TOFU

Will-Pak Foods, Inc.
1448 240th St.
Harbor City, CA 90710
800-874-0883

* **Wisdom of the Ancients**
640 S. Perry Lane
Tempe, AZ 85281
800-899-9908

Wolf Brand Products
PO Box 802521
Dallas, TX 75380
800-414-WOLF

Woodstock Organics
126 N. Main St.
New City, NY 10956
914-634-1419

Worthington Foods, Inc.
900 Proprietors Rd.
Worthington, OH 43085
800-243-1810

* **Wow-Bow Distributors**
13B Lucon Dr.
Deer Park, NY 11729
800-326-0230

* **Wysong Medical Corp.**
1880 N. Eastman
Midland, MI 48642
800-748-0188

* **The Yogi Tea Company**
2545 Prairie Rd.
Eugene, OR 97402
800-YOGI-TEA

Yves Veggie Cuisine, Inc.
1638 Derwent Way
Delta, BC V3M 6R9
Canada 604-525-1345

Food Index

almond milk, 15
amazake, 18
babaganoush, 60
bacon, veggie, 50, 51, 54, 55
balogna, veggie, 52, 53
barbecue ribs, veggie, 51
beans, baked, 32
beans, refried, 32-33
breakfast foods, 5, 36, 37, 78, 80
brownies, 89-90
burgers, veggie, 43-47
burritos, 78, 79
butter alternatives, 70, 72
camping foods, 36-37
chai, 109
cheese, non-dairy, 19-23
chicken, veggie, 49-53, 55
chili, 26, 27, 28, 30-31, 36, 74, 75, 76
chocolate mousse, 92-93
chocolates, 90-92
chorizo, veggie, 53, 54
chutney, 58
coffee substitutes, 106-108
cookies, 93-96
corndogs, 48
couscous, 26, 27, 28, 36
creamer, non-dairy, 18
cream cheese, non-dairy, 23
dessert toppings, 97-98, 102
desserts, 36, 89-104
dips, 59-60, 87
dried fruits, 39, 40, 41
dried vegetables, 38-39, 42
dumplings, 80, 81, 88
egg rolls, 81, 88
enchiladas, 78, 79
frozen foods, 73-83, 98-100, 102-104

fruit butter, 69, 70, 71, 72
fruit gelatin, 100
graham crackers, 94, 95, 96
granola, 36
grated cheese, non-dairy, 19, 20, 21
ground-meat substitutes, 50-52
guacamole, 59-60
ham, veggie, 50-51, 53, 56
hemp foods, 21, 38, 40, 47, 62
hot chocolate, 108
hot dogs, veggie, 47-49
hummus, 59, 60
ice cream, non-dairy, 98-100
Indian food, 37, 58, 67, 74-75
international foods, 75-76
Italian food, 36, 37, 53-54, 75, 76-77
jerky, 56
kitty litter, 131-133
knishes, 78
lasagna, 76
macaroni and cheese, 34, 73
manicotti, 76, 77
margarine substitute, 70, 72
mayonnaise substitute, 70, 71
meat loaf, veggie 73, 76
meatballs, veggie, 52, 77, 88
Mexican dishes, 50, 53, 54, 78-79, 96
muffins, 5
mushroom pilaf, 36
multi-grain beveragea, 15-16
oat milk, 15
Oriental dishes, 36, 37, 75, 76, 79-81, 87-88
pâté, 86-87
peanut butter, 36, 71
pepperoni, veggie, 51, 54, 55, 56

pet food, 124-130
pierogies, 88
pies, 101
pizza, 81-82
pocket meals, 83
pot pies, 73, 74, 83
potato-based milk substitutes,
    16, 17
powdered milk substitutes, 16-17
preserves, 69, 71, 72
pretzels, 38, 90, 91, 94
pudding, 101-102
ramen, 26, 29
ravioli, 77
relish, 61
rice and beans, 26, 27, 28, 29,
    33, 36, 76
rice milk, 13-14
romanelli, veggie, 53
salad dressing, 61-64
salsa, 64-66
samosas, 75
sandwich meats, veggie, 52-53
sausage, veggie, 50, 51, 53-55
sauces, 62, 66-68
scones, 102
seasoning sprays, 69
seitan, 55
shakes, 18-19
shepherd's pie, 73
Sloppy Joe, 55, 67
smoothies, 15, 19
snack foods, 36, 38-42, 56
sorbet, 102-104
soups, 25-29, 36
sour cream substitute, 23
soynut butter, 70, 72
soy milk, 10-13
spreads, 61, 69-72, 87
stevia, 110, 117-122

stew, 29, 76
stuffed cabbage, 76
sweeteners, 117-122
tamales, 79, 96
tea, 108-110
tempeh burgers, 46-47
terrine, 86
tofu burgers, 47
tofu, smoked, 87
tuna, veggie, 56
turkey, veggie 49, 52-53, 85-86
veggie wrap, 77, 83
wild rice pilaf, 36
wontons, 87
yogurt, non-dairy, 24

About the Author

Gail Davis is a nutritional consultant, speaker and author of *The Complete Guide to Vegetarian Convenience Foods*, which is the new and updated version of the original edition, (NewSage Press) as *So, Now What Do I Eat*. Her newspaper column "Eat your Vegetables!" appears regularly in the Albuquerque Weekly Alibi.

A vegetarian for more than a decade, she has interviewed many prominent physicians, scientists and nutritional experts and written about the relationship between our food choices and their impact on human health.

Davis teamed up with New Jersey physician Robert Baker, and successfully fought for the passage of legislation concerning the prevention of breast cancer. The bill requires doctors in New Jersey to supply patients with a pamphlet describing the connection between diet and breast cancer.

Davis lives in Albuquerque, New Mexico with her feline companion, Indiana Jones, and canine companion, Cicely Alaska, both confirmed vegetarians.

**For more information on other books
published by NewSage Press:**

http://www.teleport.com/~newsage

NewSage Press
phone (503) 695-2211
fax (503) 695-5406
email newsage@teleport.com